Changing
My Perspective

REBECCA S MEADOWS

Changing My Perspective

Copyright ©2020 by REBECCA S MEADOWS

ISBN: 978-1-7349947-5-9 (Paperback)
ISBN: 978-1-7349947-6-6 (Kindle Mobi)
ISBN: 978-1-7349947-7-3 (ePub)
ISBN: 978-1-7349947-8-0 (Ingram)
ISBN: 978-1-7349947-9-7 (Audible)

Edited by Johanna Petronella Leigh

Published by BLUE BUTTERFLY ENTERPRISES, LLC

Chapter 1

As I opened the door of the Missoula County courthouse on my way out that dreary January day in 2012, I had no inclination of what would happen next in my life. All I knew for sure at that moment in time was that I had finally won my freedom. I wanted to run like hell to get away from the courthouse before the judge changed his mind. I'd been living under the tyranny of the whims of various judges since the lawsuit was initially filed when I was a child and I'd had enough of it!

The guardianship was supposed to "protect" me from myself and strangers. Instead; because of the way it had initially been administered, I wound up feeling awfully naked and defiled. Once I defeated it, I felt like a fugitive from justice. I was literally terrified of being seen and recognized by the wrong person and then dragged back into court.

This reaction seems typical for someone who has been released from captivity or slavery. Why was I experiencing these emotions then? How does a young woman who has been deemed to be in need of protection become the victim of such treachery? Worse, why was it being perpetrated upon her by the very people who were supposed to be protecting her? Why had the guardianship become my adversary?

I'll tell you . . . because of the ill-conceived way in which guardianships are currently being administered in this country. Far too much emphasis is put on protecting the material possessions of the ward, often because the guardian has some design on gaining possession of them. The ward is completely helpless to do anything to stop this process once he or she has been deemed "incapacitated."

It's the most unbelievable phenomenon I've ever seen. You are suddenly transformed from a human being to something akin to a burnt-out lamp sitting on an end table the instant that judge's gavel comes down and pronounces your sentence. Everything you say is suddenly regarded as completely irrelevant—even by those who are supposed to "love" you.

This is the very situation in which all four of my parents turned away from me . . . so I know what I'm talking about.

The overwhelming sense of abandonment that filled my being the moment I realized my new situation . . . it was chilling! I felt like everything I had tried to accomplish up to that point in my life had been rendered down to nothing.

From the very moment I awoke to discover I was blind as a young girl it had always been there in the back of my mind; this urgent feeling that *I just had to overcome to live independently. I couldn't fathom the idea of being dependent upon or vulnerable to others for the rest of my life, especially my parents! There was simply no other option for me.* I refused to allow my blindness to prevent me from living a complete life!

When my parents did this to me, suddenly there I was—back at square one. I had to prove not only that I *could* live my life; but that I was willing to live it according to the dictates of others.

There were my four parents; all far away from me, a guardian who was also far away and equipped with a suspicious mind, a manipulative case manager and a neuropsychologist who had been treating me for the wrong type of brain injury for years and years—all of them trying to run *my* life. Worst of all; *their* agenda was protecting my assets from me! It was ridiculous! I dreamed for so many years of the day when I would be allowed to make my own decisions. To be honest, I was doubtful whether that day would ever come.

Sitting here at my desk writing this, I still half expect to awaken and discover I'm trapped in the nightmare yet again. Will I ever feel totally secure again? I can only hope . . .

Walking out of court that day . . . it felt like being released from prison; a prison without walls. I had been searching for the way out for so long. And I finally found it!

As you can probably imagine; it's been very difficult to voluntarily return to a courthouse.

This has greatly affected my ability to get anything legal accomplished. Imagine trying to avoid these large public structures as an adult? Thank God I never get traffic citations!

My parents' little escapade truly devastated my sense of personal security. I knew instinctively what I was capable of but convincing them of this proved nearly impossible. What can you do though? You can keep trying to live or roll over and die.

I spent so many wasted years beating my head against a brick wall. It was ridiculous; trying to convince someone to give me a chance to simply live my life in peace.

Taking someone's rights away when they're already going through a rough patch in life is like seeing someone on the ground who needs to be helped up and then deciding it's a good idea to kick them in the teeth before bending down to offer assistance. What kind of person does this? My jaw throbs every time I remember life with my parents. They loved "kicking me in the teeth."

I long ago forgave the doctor who started this whole thing. I, however, can't get over what my own parents did. The doctor was acting with a pure intention; he did not set out to harm me. What my own parents did to me so many years later though, was done intentionally and so they could diminish my personal value even further. How do I come to terms with this? I'm still trying to figure it out . . .

Legal technicalities aside, I believe there was outright corruption in the way my case was handled. Both judges who oversaw my guardianship were friends with Pete. Right then and there they should have recused themselves from my case. I'm not certain how the judge would have ruled on my petition to terminate in 2012 when I finally won my freedom had Vern not also been a friend of his.

I remember my attorney pointing out the strategy of presenting Vern to the judge in 2004 as an alternate guardian because of his well-known friendship with the judge. Does this sound like a good reason to hire someone to manage someone else's life . . . because of his or her alliances?

Of course not! This is what you get when there is this level of corruption in the government though. I'm just glad my attorney was able to manipulate the system in my favor this last time. This is not how our system works best to keep all of us safe though and people need to think about this. What are these judges doing who we've elected? Are they doing their jobs or are they just helping out their buddies from the bench whenever possible? Obviously, there needs to be some accountability in our judicial system.

Putting my life and affairs in the hands of two crooks whose only concern had always been getting their hands on the money in question seems to be pretty ridiculous to me. Pete and Joanne only wanted to conserve the money for themselves and Becca be damned! This was clearly a recipe for disaster. Perhaps the money needed a guardian, but I required something more. I was in desperate need of someone who actually cared more about my welfare than my material possessions. Sadly, this was not a reasonable expectation of my own mother or her friend Pete; the two people who'd said in the beginning they were only interested in my welfare and this was why they were suing the government. It's really appalling; the way they used a blind child to get so much money from the feds.

Can you imagine trying to find someone to handle my affairs for me who would not be more interested in the money than my well-being? By grace, Vern was available and willing to take this position in my life. I can definitely see the hand of God in this one. Vern had just the right amount of compassion and intelligence to handle the job.

The day I met Vern in his office for the first time I was a blubbering mess. I had just lost my first bid to get my constitutional rights and property restored to me and it was a rough brawl in court. I had, of course, fought very, very hard and was shocked when I was unsuccessful. All I was trying to do was get access to what most other Americans take for granted, right? How could I possibly lose? It seemed pretty cut and dried to my attorneys and me.

Imagine my shock when the judge uttered those words, *"Motion to terminate is denied!"* I felt like the judge had just kicked me in the teeth. I remember the thought crossing my mind . . . *what's wrong with you that even this judge thinks you're too stupid to manage your life?*

Then, during his closing statements for the record, the judge stated he was concerned about protecting the money. This was his reason for choosing to rule against me.

Can you believe that shit? I was incensed, to say the least.

Right from the judge's big mouth. Like I've been saying for years now, the legal and judicial systems in Montana are full of hidden corruption.

This was when I realized I had to figure out how to manipulate the system against itself. It was stacked against me. My only option was to fight back.

I had dealt with discrimination based on my blindness before but never from elected officials and it truthfully hurt. It felt like *the whole world* was stacked against me. Where could I turn for relief?

These experiences in court where I was dehumanized by both my parents and my government have made me a stronger person. When no one has your back; that's when you pull yourself up by your bootstraps and take care of business on your own.

The good old boy mentality that permeates the legal and judicial system throughout the state of Montana just drives me crazy! How is a person supposed to get a fair trial there? What happened to law and justice? Apparently, they no longer matter when you're friends with the judge.

I finally had to accept it and go on with life; there was nothing else to do. I'm afraid I was still a bit naive about how the world works.

I remember when I was on the witness stand in 2004 giving my testimony to the judge under Shannon Daniel's *brutal* cross-examination. Daniels was the lawyer for the bank. I knew him for years because he "represented" my mother in various court proceedings. He clung to the coattails of my account for as long as he could—milking me for every cent he could get out of me. Each time my account would change hands to a different administrator he would change clients to represent the person or entity who was now in control of it. He was like a blood-sucking leach. Isn't that strange? It really looked to me like he was keeping his hand buried deep in my pocket as long as he could.

As I sat upon the witness stand, Daniels handed me a document; insisting I read it aloud for the entire courtroom to hear, knowing I was incapable of such a feat. I struggled to hold back tears of humiliation as I stared up at him and admitted I was unable to read it. I was shocked I was being treated so rudely by this lawyer. My visual impairment was a well-documented fact and was not in question in the hearing. The only reason he had for doing this to me was to make sport of me in front of everyone and the judge allowed it to go on! I absolutely despised that man. I finally managed to have him fired in 2004. That was essentially the first thing I did when I finally rid myself of Pete, I fired his cronies; Shannon, Marjory and Harris. I felt it was time to get some people in place who were working *on my behalf* rather than against me. Of course, I wasn't the person who in reality gave them the notice they were terminated but it felt awesome all the same.

I was just doing the calculations in my mind as I was writing this passage. Daniels, Pete and Joanne were allowed by the government to have unfettered access to my life and account for 12 years by the time I finally ran them off in 2004. How sick is that? It makes me so angry to realize this today.

I would like to take this opportunity to make a few additional points I think are quite valid. This runaway legal mess I found myself trapped in was such a farce. First, the reason for it was to protect my money, right? Why give it to the crooks who were so greedy for it in the first place and trust them to protect it for me? The amount of waste and abuse that went on when Pete was guardian was downright appalling! It still makes me so angry. I feel like the government tied my hands and then let a bunch of thieves come into my home and just walk off with my property while I was forced to sit back and watch. Why was this permitted? This still stymies me. Second, the entire point was to allegedly protect me, right? After the judge was done with me in 1997, he washed his hands of me and I was chopped liver from that day forward—he didn't care to follow up on my situation any further. If judges are going to be permitted to screw with people's lives in such a dramatic fashion as this, they should have to follow the person's life until they either release them from the bondage or they make sure the person is still in a good situation. Pete should not have been allowed to abuse all of us the way he did. I'm so angry the state of Montana just set him upon me like a rabid dog and left him there to wreak such havoc in my life for so long; completely unrestrained and unsupervised.

When I realized my rights were gone; what was left to live for? My fate was in the hands of others.

It has taken me several years to understand what went wrong in court that night in 1997 to cause this runaway legal mess in my life. I believe I've figured it out.

When my parents set out to protect the money instead of me there was a shift in the intention of the events in court that night. Suddenly I was the focus of the hearing in word only. As the money was elevated— so I was demoted. This subtle change of intention rendered me worthless. In everyone's heart, the true purpose became to protect the *money*. I was merely an afterthought in the whole thing!

When the state of Montana stripped me of my constitutional rights and then turned me over to Pete the way they did, this left me completely defenseless to everyone—including my parents. Does this sound like a way to "guard" a person? It was all bass-ackwards.

How can a guardianship that is set up to protect one's property from one's self ever succeed? This makes the ward the suspect, not the one in need of protection. That's the foundation the guardianship was founded upon. It was doomed from its conception. As someone who experienced this ridiculousness firsthand; perhaps I'm qualified to offer a solution?

If the ward were to maintain all their rights, specifically the right to receive counsel on how to manage their affairs, I believe situations such as this could be resolved much quicker. And with far less financial and emotional hardship on their family. Isn't that the actual goal of guardianships? Giving the individual their dignity and control over their destiny Wow, sounds like a radical idea, don't you think?

I remember the sick feeling that settled in the pit of my stomach as I was led from the courtroom that night in 1997. I knew I was totally screwed. My only comfort was my young age; perhaps someday I would be able to rectify this injustice so I could live my life. I had no idea it would take 15 exhausting years to accomplish it!

I remember when I met Vern for the first time in 2004. I was hesitant to agree to the idea of presenting him to the judge as an alternate guardian because of his advanced years. I quickly realized with him as my guardian, this could wind up being the avenue God would use to eventually release me from the guardianship. He very well might just expire while in office and I would be free. I realized long ago the right hand of the government rarely knows what the left hand is doing.

Looking back; I'm appalled at how I felt about Vern that day when I first met him. I was looking forward to his eventual demise so I could be free. He eventually became one of my most ardent supporters. If it hadn't been for him; I would have never escaped.

I think that judge—the first one, the one in Havre that night in 1997—bears the most responsibility in all of this. He's the one who stripped me of my property and constitutional rights with such little regard for me. He's the one who set the guardianship up in this manner. Last I heard that genius had been appointed to sit on the supreme court in Montana. Can you believe that? This judge was the first one to violate my constitutional rights. The other judge, the one in Missoula in 2004, was just signing off on what looked like a foregone conclusion.

If he had simply done his job and *protected me and my* constitutional rights at that initial hearing or even at the next one six months later;

this all could have been avoided. This is why I feel so strongly the laws need to be changed to guarantee protection to others!

I realized when I was first going through this process back in 2003 there was quite a bit of malignancy; if you will, in the foundation of the guardianship. It just wasn't set up correctly. I remember telling people, "The guardianship just 'broke.'" I thought *I* broke it. Now, with all I have learned, I can clearly see it was a corrupt deal from the beginning. This will continue to happen to other innocent people until the rights of the ward are truly protected.

I remember the sick feeling that rose up inside me when I realized the size and scope of what I was facing. It felt like an insurmountable task, redirecting everyone's attention off of the shiny object and back onto me. How was I going to accomplish this?

I felt incredibly weary as I was coming to this realization. Life had already been so challenging . . . did I have it in me to move *another* mountain?

This has been a life-altering experience that has consumed literally thirty years of my life. I had no inkling that day in 1989 when I opened my eyes I was about to embark on such an epic journey to recovery. My every thought and impulse since the day when this first began has been geared towards this goal of regaining my free will.

That was the whole problem. *My* agenda has *always* been different from that of everyone else involved in this "project" over the years. I'm the one who has been living in this body with this brain and am therefore the only one who knows exactly what's going on in here. I'm the only person who has a pure motive. I grew so sick of listening to doctors and lawyers telling my parents and me what I was supposedly thinking and feeling and their opinions of why I was this way. I just wanted to ask them one question back then, but I couldn't—I wasn't allowed to. *What made my parents, all the doctors and the lawyers so convinced they knew my mind better than I did?* The gall of some people!

When I finally had the chance to discuss with my mother what happened to me because of her guardianship shenanigan she made a phone call and set me free from it. What about all the years I lost before she did this though! What am I supposed to do now? I litcrally lost 15 years of my life to that guardianship! Not to mention all the financial cost and emotional trauma to my family and me. As you can clearly hear in my voice, I am a long way from forgiveness on this one. I know this is really holding me back on the remainder of my healing but I'm still trying to figure out how to just let it go.

There are several things I would like to fix about guardianships and mark my words; someday I will tackle this project. I'm not one of those people who sits around and complains about a bad situation—I like to try to make it better. I know, I may have my work cut out for me, but someone has to do it.

The ADA (Americans with Disabilities Act) wouldn't even consider taking on my case when I reached out to them for assistance in 2004. I was literally told guardianships are just too tough for them to take on. Who was I supposed to turn to for relief? What recourse do other disabled Americans have when they are told by the ADA even *they* are too weak to take on guardianships?

I had to figure out how to defeat this crazy, messed up law all alone. I pray others can find the strength to move one of these mountains on their own if they should find one in their life's path as well. Perhaps I can show them the way.

Regaining my constitutional rights so dramatically was quite a shock to my traumatized system. Fortunately, I realized what a huge change was coming in my life, so I did my best to prepare for it. The day the judge released me I was already formulating a plan in my mind for how I would try to do this without making any huge mistakes.

The best thing I could think of was to simply wait for a period of time to let the dust settle before I did anything significant with my life. To be perfectly honest, I think what I feared most back then was that I might just crack up while trying to adjust to having so much freedom. What if I pushed the wrong button on the computer of my life and it self-destructed?

Following the incident in Missoula where I was smoking marijuana with my "caregivers," I was told when preparing for the lawsuit a team of doctors had made predictions. They were supposedly educated guesses about what decisions and paths I might choose throughout life as a result of the brain damage resulting from the tumor. I was also told these mysterious predictions were coming true. When I asked to see the list, I was denied. For a long time following this experience, I felt utterly hopeless. If I were so messed up that a bunch of doctors were able to predict my mistakes so far in advance, then what was the point of trying to overcome my disability any further? Clearly, I was doomed to fail, right? Hadn't it been foretold?

For a long time, I really struggled to overcome this experience. Imagine it!

I was overwhelmed by a sense of dread when I tried to make any decision at all for fear I might make one of those fatal decisions I was warned of and something terrible would happen as a result.

I was so nervous afterward. The experience was horrible! I wondered if this meant I would always be the same failure I felt like at that point in my life. I mean, if I was so messed up that a bunch of doctors viewed me as some kind of experiment, how was I supposed to ever become something more than what they were saying I was capable of?

I woke up when I was 12 years old; just as I was about to embark on puberty—one of the most significant periods of development in a person's life. I entered this new realm with a fractured identity. As I was grappling to figure out who and what I was, everyone around me was so busy telling me who *they* decided I was allowed to be. Is it any wonder I was confused?

My parents, the lawyers and everyone else had always treated the doctors as though they were God and knew exactly what was going on so of course, I assumed the doctors were correct.

Over time, as I was becoming aware they really didn't have a clue why I said and did the things I did, I began to realize what a pickle I was in. How was I going to "prove" to all these people they were wrong about me? An even greater question: how had they become so convinced they were better at living *my* life than *I* was? They had all decided what steps they thought I should take throughout life and if I chose differently it was chalked up to another bad decision—just because my decision was different from what they wanted. My life was literally stolen from me all over again; just as it was when I first awoke from my coma! This was so very frustrating for me. Just imagine . . . your every choice is monitored and judged to see if it measures up to someone else's standards. How was I supposed to ever manage to please all these people so they would leave me alone to just live my life in peace?

As I've already pointed out; people, especially people in certain positions, need to be careful about how they phrase things to others.

The day my mother told me about the predictions and that they were coming true, I felt very hopeless.

I was dealing with my arrested childhood again. All of these "bad" decisions could easily be traced back to this single incident, but no one seemed to be taking this into account. It was really ridiculous. All those years I was regularly being told what a massive screw-up I was, but no one seemed to be interested in helping me figure out how to get better. I wonder if they genuinely didn't have a clue what they were doing so they were using me as a guinea pig? That's what it felt like . . . anyway.

That's another reason I've written my books, to try to help them figure the brain out better. Who knows? Maybe something I've shared will put them on the right track.

I was so angry when the preparations for the lawsuit were going on. My mother was able to tell her story to lots of people—both professionals and her friends. But no one wanted to know what I was thinking and feeling about what happened and I was the one it had happened to. I have waited all these years to tell my story.

I was in high school and was an avid reader of John Grisham's novels when I realized I was living a life that would one day be worthy of one of his legal thrillers. And here I am, writing it myself!

During Pete's administration, my development was quite stunted due to all the restrictions he placed in my path. Fortunately, when Vern was my guardian, he permitted me to have a much longer leash so the shock wasn't as severe as it might have been when I finally gained my freedom.

Understandably, perhaps, I still felt like I was walking through a magic portal into a completely new world as I was exiting the courthouse for the final time on that most righteous day in January of 2012.

When I awoke the following morning to start living life as a fully emancipated adult, I remember wondering how to begin this process. The feeling of giddiness was almost surreal. For the first time in my life, I could literally go anywhere and do anything I wanted to; just like everyone else. To be perfectly frank; it was an absolutely terrifying experience for me! Imagine that; for the very first time in your life, you suddenly have all this freedom. I nearly decided to hide in my bed that entire day. Frankly, the whole first year was quite interesting really.

I had lived in Missoula since 1997 and knew a lot of people who lived there. Every time I went out and someone would recognize me calling out my name from nearby, I would jump in horror. I was so very terrified of being taken against my will and shanghaied again. During all those years under the guardianship, I was keenly aware of my situation. My home in Missoula was essentially a prison without bars. I could only go so far from it without getting permission from someone else. It was similar to being under house arrest. This had gone on for most of my adult life. How can they expect a person to simply start living normally after something like that?

This will probably sound a little weird but bear with me for a moment. Another peculiar phenomenon I experienced following the termination was how I felt about Vern. I remember feeling a strong urge to turn back to him for protection. He was a much more reasonable person than Pete was. When Vern was my guardian, I knew I was safe from another attempt by my mother to regain control of my property. Now, I'm not protected from her and this still makes me feel uneasy. I

actually contemplated trying to cut a deal with Vern for continued protection from her. It's ridiculous to think the person I fear most is my
own mother but after what happened . . . can you blame me?

Once I had my rights and property returned to me, I knew I wasn't
satisfied with where my life was at that moment. It seemed like a daunt-
ing task that cold winter's day; figuring out how to make my life my own.
How does one *start* living a life that has already been constructed—and
that by the decisions and whims of so many other people? It was quite
a conundrum; most of the time people are making these kinds of decisions when they are around the age of 18 years or so but there I was, 35
years old and trying to suddenly figure out how to just get started. The
day I walked out of court I owned a house in Missoula with no mortgage
on it, but did I want to spend the rest of my life in the mountains? What
options were out there for me now that I had the freedom to pursue
them? These were only a few of the questions that weighed heavily on
my mind at that point.

In those early days, I was also terrified of doing something stupid
and losing all my money. For many years, the belief had been impressed
upon me I was not capable of handling such a large sum of cash. Suddenly it was mine to wrangle. If I were to mess up and lose it all, this
would certainly be poetic justice as far as my mother and her cronies
were concerned.

Looking back now, I'm shocked that was my main concern at the
time. Was I really ready to handle all of this? In a way, I felt unfairly
burdened; what other blind woman had to concern herself with such
things? It was then I started to understand the walls that were created
in my life by the presence of the money in my world. How was I supposed to integrate into the blind community when my friends were
always commenting on how much nicer things were in my life than
theirs simply because of the money? Like I pointed out previously, the
money didn't fix the blindness, so I simply tried to make my life more
comfortable and less stressful with it, but this didn't go unnoticed by
my peers.

I really hated what happened with the lawsuit. When it was filed, the focus was suddenly shifted from my medical care to winning the lawsuit. It was as if my mother had a new interest to throw herself at. This greatly exasperated my already tenuous situation.

My relationships at school were also dramatically affected by the lawsuit. It was so awkward being confronted all the time by other kids asking questions about my family's financial or legal situation I really couldn't and didn't want to answer. This made school even more unbearable than it already was.

If you look at the situation from my perspective; you can easily understand how I came to loathe the money that was thrust upon me as a child. I didn't ask for any of this but it's what happened. It would be nice if I could go back and change how things worked out.

Now, my life is much different. I think my current situation is much closer to what my mother envisioned for my life when she initially started all of this with her lawsuit. I am finally master of my own destiny. The money has become a tool in my life rather than a mammoth hurdle I'm constantly trying to vault over. I could have been living like this much sooner if the focus was on the correct intentions in the beginning.

This all started the moment I opened my eyes that day in 1989 to discover I was suddenly blind. As I pointed out earlier, this was a shocking and nearly crippling experience. There was so much more loss here than just the loss of physical sight. These losses were fairly easy to pin a monetary value upon. For many years now, however, the loss that grieves me the most is the loss of my relationship with my mother. She cannot see I have survived and recovered. It is as though she needs to justify her lawsuit against the federal government and if she acknowledges I am no longer a broken, worthless creature, then her lawsuit was a sham.

Let me tell you what I think happened. My mother witnessed my death in the ambulance. This is a fact. I wound up surviving but with a completely different personality than her daughter. She took me home but never did reconnect with me. This made it so much easier for her to overlook me in her quest to protect the money so many years later. I'm not a doctor but this makes sense to me when nothing else does.

I was my mother's first "little girl." She has always said she just wants her little girl back. None of us can turn back the clock. I cannot be what she wants. She doesn't want a broken daughter.

To have your mother completely wipe your very existence from her awareness . . . it's like being murdered. Then you realize you're not actually dead; *she's* the one who's dead. This is where I'm currently stuck at with my healing where my mom is concerned. Perhaps she'll learn how to live again someday.

In the coming chapters, I will show you other ways in which we are all still losing in this situation. Is there a way for me to turn this around so *someone* can score a true victory? We'll see . . .

Author's note: the day I added this passage to my manuscript, in my heart, I challenged God to help me make it so; to help me do something really incredible. It was about three months later that I met Gino.

Chapter 2

As I said before; living in Missoula was nearly impossible for me due to the trauma we all suffered there—myself in particular. Because of this, I was definitely open to the idea of getting out of dodge.

Over time I began learning about options available to someone like me through my affiliation with the NFB (National Federation of the Blind). I eventually became aware of a school in Minneapolis that was specifically designed for blind adults to receive training in Braille and other necessary skills. It was a "blind immersion" training program. I traveled to Minneapolis to check out the training center. I liked what I learned while touring the facility, so I enrolled at the school and began classes.

The school is amazing! The center is located in the old Pillsbury mansion. That place is ideal for a blind school.

I had pretty decent O&M (Orientation and Mobility) skills before I went there. Navigating that place with a sleep shade on has been one of my greatest challenges as a blind traveler. Talk about a labyrinth!

Perhaps the most astonishing feature of the Pillsbury Mansion is its "grand staircase" that engulfs a large area of the school. The entire building is bursting with great opportunities to practice your skills.

I spent so much time hopelessly lost in the basement on more than one occasion when my instructor would send me down there on O&M lessons.

I swear I could feel unseen eyes staring at me from the darkness as I nervously trudged through those echoing concrete hallways wearing my sleep shade. It was so eerie!

This was the place where I learned to cook under a sleep shade.

I never doubted my ability to cook. I just hadn't been allowed to before—not like this.

Both my mothers ordered me to stay far away from their stoves when I was a teenager when my mothers should have been teaching me to cook. Learning to do this without being able to see anything at all on both an electric and gas stove was awesome. I was scratching my head the whole time I was learning this; wondering how my mothers expected me to learn this on my own.

This was the place I learned the Braille code as well.

My relationship with Braille has been a rocky one over the years.

Braille felt like a huge, scary monster when I became blind as a child. I still don't understand why it felt so. I know my mother and others close to me were having a lot of trouble accepting the blindness and so the cane and Braille were rejected as well.

When I began my Braille studies, I noticed right away my brain latched onto the Braille code like it was a drug. It was crazy!

I would lay awake at night reviewing the Braille code in my head, rewriting conversations from school that day in Braille contractions in my mind. It was like my brain couldn't stop thinking in Braille. My brain felt like it was buzzing. I hadn't experienced this since I went to Bridges.

Before my TBI (Traumatic brain injury) rehab training, I experienced this crazy insomnia for years that acted a lot like this.

Do you want to know what I think as the one who lived through it? I think my brain was buzzing after the brain injury. I think my brain had so much trouble slowing down because I was extremely smart before the tumor. I think the tumor incident sent my brain into a sort of tantrum. It felt like I had a very severe case of ADHD in my brain.

When I went to Bridges, I found immediate relief from this. It surfaced again years later when my brain was in a position to think a lot.

I've been experiencing something similar to this again recently since I opened my company. That story comes much later. For now, I just want to say I believe my brain still wanted to think and was trying desperately to do so with all that buzzing. It would literally go until I blacked out.

My brain's response to learning Braille was such a shock to me. When I tried to learn Braille right after the injury, I couldn't do it. I think it was the fact I received my TBI rehab training years before this that changed the ball game for me.

I actually know one other thing that stood in my way back in the beginning: grief.

When they tried to force Braille on me, I was still grieving and was not ready to tackle it. They only tried that first summer and only for a week at the summer orientation program the MAB (Montana Association for the Blind) used to put on back then.

I suspect if I had received support from my parents and teachers with learning Braille, I would have been able to learn it much earlier.

Thank God I found the NFB when I did. I only wish my parents had stumbled upon them for me when I was a kid.

When I joined the NFB after I dissolved the guardianship, I found their philosophy echoed what I had always believed about myself and had been trying to prove for years.

That is; blind people can do anything; blindness is not what holds us back.

While at the facility, I cheated on my husband with a fellow blind student who I met there.

My husband forgave me. At the time, he picked up everything and moved himself and our children to Minneapolis to live with me.

While in Minneapolis we rented a house located near the MSP international airport.

Life in that domicile was very trying for all of us; myself most of all. It was ridiculously small and cramped. We didn't know any of our neighbors and we occasionally heard gunshots in our neighborhood.

The noises of the jets when they flew low over the house as they were taking off or coming in for a landing were absolutely terrifying for me. I was probably quite a bit more sensitive to it than my husband and children because of my enhanced hearing, but I'm quite certain they were also very unhappy with our circumstances.

I remember all our clothes and other possessions reeked of jet fuel when we lived there. This substance smells like kerosene. As a blind person, the entire experience living in that house in Minneapolis was a nightmare.

During that time, I was counting the months until we could leave.

It wasn't all bad, living in Minnesota; that is. We spent a lot of time getting to know my dad and stepmother who lived nearby. We were driving north to spend time with them nearly every weekend. They also came to our house in Minneapolis. I had the opportunity to get reacquainted with some of my more distant relations who lived throughout Minnesota as well. It was great!

While at the school, I learned the Braille code and how to use the JAWS (Job Access With Speech) program to operate a computer better. I also learned how to do many things under a sleep shade. My trust in my cane grew exponentially during this time as well. There is definitely something to be said about the benefits of taking vision out of the equation.

It was while returning to our home in Minneapolis after I'd gone to an NFB convention out of state that it happened.

As the plane approached the MSP airport I was suddenly overcome by an oppressive shroud. I felt an overwhelming need to get away from this man I had married. I actually found myself contemplating suicide as an alternative to going home to him! I realized right away this wasn't good. If I was *this* unhappy, I needed to make a change. I had been dissatisfied for a long time but had felt trapped and unable to do anything about it because of the restraints of the guardianship. Now that it was gone, it was time to put on my big girl pants and make a decision one way or the other. Was I going to stay in a loveless marriage, or could I find the strength to walk away?

I looked back at the entirety of my life. I thought about my early childhood, before the tumor. I reflected upon those early years following it when I was a lonely teenager. I recalled the arguments I'd had with my mother and stepmother. I thought about how I was railroaded into that guardianship. I remembered what it felt like to finally get the treatment I received at Bridges. I remembered when I was being forced to pay for LST (Life Skills Trainers)s to sit in my home and monitor my activities while documenting everything I was doing.

I also thought about everything I had learned as a married woman and mother.

I figured if God had arranged for all this unique training in my life, He must have a pretty important job for me to do while I'm here so there was no time to lose. I could plainly see I was just spinning my wheels. What was I doing? I knew I had to make a change sooner rather than later. I had already lost fifteen years of my life. It suddenly felt like I didn't have much left to live.

Chapter 3

I had been half-heartedly looking for a second home in a warmer climate for a while. Since we were uprooted from our home in Missoula it seemed like it might be a good time to get more serious about our search.

I was considering Florida as a possible location but after Jeff Bush was swallowed alive by that sinkhole, I changed my mind in a hurry!

I had already experienced many anomalies in life. First, the tumor. Then there was the lawsuit settlement. This was *actually* deemed a "historic" event in the history of the state of Montana. I was then railroaded into that stupid guardianship—also a very bizarre situation. Then I just happened to meet my husband, a man who also survived some pretty hairy medical mistakes before I met him. We came together and created two children, both of whom have been unique in their own ways. Then there were the two court battles to regain my constitutional rights and property from the state of Montana.

After all of this, I felt certain I would be asking for trouble moving to Florida. I didn't want to become the first person to be swallowed alive by a sinkhole who managed to climb out!

My husband had free time on his hands while we were living in Minneapolis, so I assigned him the task of finding us a second home. I sent him to Arizona to look.

He was originally from Arizona and we visited there a few times during our marriage, so I knew I liked the environment. He made several trips down there to meet with a real estate agent to look at prospective homes while the children and I attended our classes in Minneapolis.

We eventually found the ideal home in Mesa and I purchased it in April of 2015. Since the kids were still finishing up the school year in Minneapolis, we didn't move to our new home right away. Once the kids were done, we moved back to Missoula temporarily.

In June of that year, I was involved in my fourth car accident while we were still in Missoula. It was largely due to the first three accidents that I felt justified in looking for a second home in a warmer climate. The fourth one just convinced me, even more, I really did need to leave my home.

That summer while Randi and the children waited back in Missoula, I made several trips to Mesa to get the new house ready for all of us to move into. I repainted the interior. I laid new carpet throughout the house and purchased new appliances and furniture. When we moved in that fall, I wanted it to be all ready for my family.

From the moment I told my husband I wanted to begin looking for a second home, there was never any question about what we would do with Mom. My mother-in-law would be going with us! We all moved to Mesa together.

Pat was a beautiful woman. She was the one who introduced me to Randi. When he eventually asked me to marry him, her first response was to inform him she was certain I was a demon and would surely steal his children from him! Isn't that hilarious?

Pat tried to sow discord in our marriage for a long time. It was amazing how much patience and grace God gave me for her. I remember the turning point in our relationship; the day she went from criticizing me to treating me like a daughter.

We were on the phone together. She was being her crotchety old self as usual. I was feeling like a heel because of whatever it was she was barraging me about. Once I was able to get a word in edgewise, I just opened my mouth, and something popped out I didn't intend. I was mortified! I was dismissive of her thoughts and feelings. She simply cleared her throat and hesitated just a moment before hanging up the phone without another word. She seemed to be quite shocked I stood up to her. I remember telling my husband about it later after I noticed she was treating me better. He warned me not to get comfortable; he was certain she would once again turn on me. Pat never did. We became much closer from then on. I guess she just needed to realize I wasn't going to allow her to treat me like a doormat any longer.

Pat needed knee replacement surgery for a while. When we decided to move to Mesa, she opted to wait and have the surgery there. She was looking forward to recovering from her surgery in the beautiful climate in Arizona.

Mom had her surgery. Then she was moved to a rehab center here in Mesa to assist her with her recovery. The center opted to take her off of a prescription-strength medication her regular doctor put her on for her IBS (irritable bowel syndrome). They put her on a cheaper, less potent drug. This new drug wasn't strong enough to fight her IBS. She wound up with C-diff. They transferred her back to the hospital to get it under control.

While in the hospital, Mom contracted pneumonia and we lost her on April 2nd, 2016.

I remember feeling like an orphan all over again. She was the only mother I'd known since I was 12 years old. I was like a big baby, crying all the time. I could still hear the echo of her laughter and the clicking of her knee echoing through my home. She used to talk about all the things she would do now that she was in Mesa once her surgery was out of the way. All those dreams which Randi and I shared with her, died that day just so that the rehab center could save a buck! This pissed me off.

Randi and I were so distraught over what happened to mom. We talked about suing the damn rehab center. What was the point though? We couldn't get Mom back.

It was her essence we were so desperately missing.

For so many nights afterward, I would be lying awake, thinking about Mom. Randi would awaken and we would wind up talking about her until the next thing I knew, we would be in each other's arms again, bawling like a couple of oversized kids! It was such a devastating blow to us.

Chapter 4

When I came to Mesa, I had to find treatment for my injuries from that last car accident. I also needed access to reliable information. So, I joined the local chapter of the NFB.

I also asked around about a good massage therapist. A couple of people suggested I try a local massage school where I could see newly graduated students for a lower price. I started my treatments there.

Over time, one of the therapists kept telling me he felt I could get better care from someone he referred to as his "mentor." I foolishly blew him off for months. It wasn't until just before Christmas when I couldn't get in to see him that I finally called his mentor.

The first time I saw Lancelot I was amazed! Having been in so many car accidents, I received massage therapy from several different therapists over the years. This guy definitely had a gift. I continued to see him and never again went back to the school for massage.

Lancelot was an amazing practitioner with a vast skill set he utilized when he worked with me. He incorporated many of these gifts over time. He used a variety of massage techniques, as well as reiki and hypnotherapy. He did a form of "yoga therapy" with me that has helped a great deal to correct long-standing inconsistencies throughout my body that have been causing me a lot of difficulties since my original injuries.

He also practiced life coaching on me. I believe this is *the tool* that has truly enabled me to change my life.

From the moment I awoke in the hospital at the tender age of 12 years old all I heard from everyone in my sphere was I couldn't do anything right anymore. This sudden turnaround in the feedback I was getting from those around me had a profound impact on me. It confused me. It frustrated me. I couldn't understand why everyone had suddenly decided I was worthless. This new reality absolutely terrified me!

I still knew deep inside I was a valid person.

After so many years of hearing variations of this mantra, it became like brainwashing. By the time I finally met my life coach I was so bound up inside I no longer had the ability to conceive of a future for myself.

This is what Lancelot did for me that I find so compelling! He helped me regain the ability to *dream*; something I was unable to do since this had all began.

From the time I awoke from that coma; I felt so strange. It was like I slipped out of my body and only partially climbed back in or like I was in but not straight. My entire being felt awfully heavy in those early years. It felt like I was lugging around someone else's body that was too large for me. At the same time, my mind and heart were barely hanging on also. I truly think my entire being, physical and otherwise, was trapped between life and death after the events in 1989.

Lancelot helped me bring it all back together. The way I felt as I was going through this process, I can only compare it to how it felt going through Bridges. Similar to the way my brain started to awaken in Bridges; the process of unlocking my heart had begun.

Lancelot was certainly not cheap. I paid his fees without complaint though. This man helped me finish the process of recovering—something no one else was able to do.

I was still quite "broken" when I met him. Then, I felt myself getting stronger every single day! I felt my being coming back online. This money was awarded to me because of what happened, so I figured I would use it to try to make myself better. I dare say; it's about time!

Chapter 5

When I joined the NFB I immediately had access to tons of information about what was available here in the Phoenix area. This worked well for me.

I had been contemplating the idea of getting my first guide dog for a while. When I came to Arizona, it seemed like it might be the right time to move on this plan as well.

One of the biggest reasons I'd shied away from getting a dog previously was because I didn't relish the idea of having to take the dog outside in the dead of winter to go to the bathroom in Montana. The climate here in Arizona is completely different though.

I began the process of checking into a guide dog. I first studied the locations of the service dog schools I was hearing about from my friends in the NFB. I immediately shied away from the ones located in areas of the country where it snowed. By this time, I realized I prefer warm weather.

I applied to a school in nearby California. Part of the application process called for a form to be filled out by an O&M instructor regarding my skill level using my cane.

I certainly wasn't concerned about whether my cane skills were good enough; I knew I had excellent skills because I use my cane all the time and *never* use a human guide. I didn't know a single orientation and mobility instructor here in Arizona though. How was I going to get this information I needed?

Again, I turned to my friends in the NFB for information.

Someone suggested I call vocational rehabilitation services.

I long ago signed up for the Voc Rehab program in Montana with no results. Would I experience something different here?

When I called, I was told in no uncertain terms I would only receive services from them if I met two qualifications. First, I had to be at least legally blind and second, I had to have a true desire to go to work because they would be putting me to work.

What? Wait just a minute! I had always been told I was incapable of working.

I felt like I had just been hit by a bus. I was in shock. Imagine hearing this after so many years of being told just the opposite? You better believe I signed up in a hurry. Then I went on Facebook and posted my announcement.

I wanted the whole world to know someone believed in me!

In high school, my teachers tried to administer an interests exam to me. During the test, a person read a list of occupations to me. Before the list was read, I was told I was supposed to rate each of the jobs based on how interested I might be in learning more about them. It was emphasized to me I was *not* to consider my blindness as a factor in any of my decisions—simply if I would like to learn more about the position.

I was elated! Finally, someone believed in me. This would be easy for me. I had been figuring out workarounds to do everything in life for so long; I felt certain my blindness would not impact my test results.

What did influence them, was the attitude of the people administering the exam to me. Each and every time I would rate a job high the exam administrator felt in her own mind I couldn't or shouldn't attempt as a blind person, she emphatically informed me of it! She eventually became so frustrated with me, she stormed out of the room in disgust having left the exam unfinished.

Believe me, she wasn't the only one in the room that day who was angry.

By this time, I had had enough of this stupidity. It had been going on for years and *I* definitely wasn't the one with the problem; everyone else was. The next person they sent in to "set me straight" didn't do any better. How was I supposed to do my part with people who thought like that? Every answer I gave was automatically wrong because *they* had decided I couldn't do anything at all. How stupid was that? I was literally the only person who believed from the very beginning I would eventually climb out of this sinkhole that had manifested in my life. Everyone was so busy shoveling the dirt back over my head whenever I managed to make any progress towards climbing out.

I was told by several of my friends I shouldn't expect anything different from VR (Vocational Rehabilitation) here either. They had all been there with VR themselves and seemed to feel they were let down. Would my experience be any different?

After a few weeks, I received a phone call from my VR counselor inviting me to participate in a week-long workshop they had scheduled for the first week of March. I signed up.

During that week, the other participants and I were introduced to several of the training centers for the blind here in the Phoenix area. I was fascinated by what I was learning. Why didn't we have training centers for blind adults in Montana? I realized why the hands of VR in Montana were tied when it came to finding reliable services for blind adults. How frustrating that must be!

By the end of the week, I knew without a doubt which of the training centers I wanted to attend. It was easy. Only one of the facilities echoed my passion for ultimate independence.

Not surprising perhaps, it was the school that had a reputation for following the NFB's militant logic on matters.

I went home after the workshop ended and waited to see what would happen next.

Within a week or so I received another call from my counselor wanting to know what I'd thought of the workshop. I excitedly told her which of the programs I wanted to attend. She put me on the waiting list.

I was a student at the center by that August.

Chapter 6

In order to begin my services with VR, I had to select a job goal. What did I want to do for the rest of my life that I would enjoy? This philosophy shocked me. People doing what they wanted for employment instead of having to settle for whatever they could get. What a novel idea! Coming from where I did, I certainly felt privileged.

Well, I knew I was great at word processing and I had been previously trained on how to use a Dictaphone. I also enjoyed talking on the phone and meeting new people. I knew I had good social skills and a warm, inviting personality that would make me an asset to any office.

To me, this spelled out just one thing . . . an administrative assistant of some kind. I told my counselor what I selected. She wrote it in my plan. I was told I would likely change my job goal several times during the process; most other people did. I was not concerned. I usually knew my mind.

I started my training.

That July, before I began my training at the school, I went to the NFB convention in Florida alone. I again engaged in acts contrary to my vows to my husband.

It was about a month later when I finally told Randi I wanted a divorce. I was certain by then I was extremely unhappy. Why else couldn't I stay faithful?

I had been watching miserable people for most of my life. People who weren't strong enough to just walk away. It was like they had just given up on life. I didn't want to wind up like them. Like I said earlier, I only had so much life left to live.

More on that later . . . I promise.

Attending the training center was incredible! All the people who were affiliated with the program shared my philosophy of life as a blind person. I no longer had to constantly fight for equal access as before. It was so refreshing!

I truly believe my parents did me a huge disservice by refusing to allow me to embrace my blindness from the very beginning. When I was terrified of it, I was in bondage to it. It was only through embracing my blindness and learning to live with it that I finally overcame it. Think about it?

Honestly, I hold the "professionals" who were in my life back then much more accountable for what happened than my poor parents. My parents didn't understand what was happening. The most any of my parents had was a high school diploma and the "professionals" were claiming they had it all figured out. Why didn't any of them help my parents understand the importance of acknowledging the situation rather than pretending it didn't exist? How differently my life may have turned out if someone had!

Many years ago, at one of the last functions I participated in with my family, we were posing for a family photo. I was standing on the end of the back row because I'm the tallest member of my family. My mother approached me, casually removing my cane from my grasp. She walked out of the area, sticking my cane in a corner somewhere. She was so ashamed of me she didn't want anyone viewing the photo later to see my cane and realize I was blind.

This act killed me! That was the day I realized my mother could no longer see me for a human being past the blindness. Did I really have to choose between a relationship with my mother *or* my own safety and independence? I knew what my answer had to be. That day my dream of reconciling with my mother died.

In 2004, when my mother testified against me in court, I finally realized the truth.

She was on the witness stand carrying on about how she just wanted her little girl back. I recalled she had been saying those very words for years in all those stupid meetings. When I realized my mother was mentally stuck back in 1989, I knew I was in deep trouble. By then I had learned my mother held the keys to my freedom from the guardianship. If she couldn't comprehend the fact I had grown up, how was I ever going to convince the state of Montana I should be emancipated?

From the time I started my training, I was hearing mysterious rumors about the computer every student eventually received. People acted like it was the Holy Grail.

I was mystified. I had a computer I had been using to write my second book for a while. When I found out I would be getting a new one that would be far superior in quality, I simply rehomed the one I was using so someone else could use it. I was going to be getting a new one that would be far superior after all.

Months and months went by with no new computer. I was panicking. I wasn't making any progress on my new book.

Then in one of my staffings at school, I pointed out to my counselor if I had a computer at home, I would be able to practice all the things they were teaching me in school. I was blown away when she turned to me and said, "I agree with you. I'll get you your computer right away." I think my mouth fell open. That afternoon I listened to a voice message from her confirming what she said in my meeting that morning. I almost burst out laughing the next day when my "boss" at school came to me bragging that because of what *he* had done, I would be getting my computer in a matter of weeks instead of some unknown date in the distant future.

It was only because I advocated for myself, not because of anything he did. The school only tried to convince us we were helpless in the process. I simply decided I wasn't going to be helpless any longer.

I received my computer from Vocational Rehabilitation a few weeks later—just before we were all scheduled to leave for the NFB convention in Florida that summer.

I worked with that machine for nearly a year and a half and had no end of headaches with it. It crashed all the time. I nearly lost my book several times during the process. My tech teacher at school helped me pull it back from the brink on several occasions.

Then a different teacher and I engaged in a yelling match because the stress of dealing with the computer became so bad. I went home after school that day very disturbed. What was I going to do? I knew I couldn't allow this situation to continue to evolve this way.

I was friends with many of my teachers at school and didn't want this crazy situation to affect our friendships. It wasn't any of our fault this was happening. Our hands were tied. I realized VR had dropped the ball.

When I signed up for VR services, they said they would provide training, reliable and accessible equipment and transportation to and from the training center if I did my part and participated fully. *I had been doing my part. VR had not.*

I sat down and emailed my counselor. I didn't mince words. I was bold. I was assertive. I told him how I saw the situation. I informed him in no uncertain terms I was only willing to participate in this fiasco for two more weeks and if he didn't get me a new computer that worked, I would not attend another class at school. Then I copied my boss at school and my tech teacher in it. I went to bed that night feeling secure in the knowledge I had done my very best to advocate for myself in this situation.

Then on my way to school the next morning, I suddenly realized it was likely I had another staffing that day. My heart skipped a beat. I would be trapped in a little room with my VR counselor, my boss at school and my tech teachers. OMG! I realized perhaps I should have held off a bit longer on my "big stand-up-for-myself email" the day before. What would happen in my meeting?

When I walked into the room, I was shocked to find one of the higher-up administrators at school sitting there. My blood ran cold. Surely, they were going to give me the boot. I nervously took my seat at the table.

The big boss looked at me and asked me what had been going on. I struggled to hold back my tears of anxiety as I began to describe to her what had been going on and how I was feeling about it.

I could see the empathy pouring from her; so acute was her support for me. I was touched.

She turned to my voc rehab counselor and asked him what could be done. He responded. Basically, now that I had made my needs known, they were going to do whatever they needed to do in order to continue to support me. He apologized there was a breakdown in communication and he had not realized we were having so much trouble with the computer. I was so moved at the level of support I felt that day. I had gone into that room terrified and come out victorious.

They said they would get me a new computer, but it could take up to two months . . . was I willing to wait? I thought about it for a moment. No, it wasn't okay. I had already lost nearly two years of time working on my new book because I listened to promises from others. They offered me access to computers at school and assistance from my teachers if I wanted it while I waited for the computer to arrive.

I could see how much they were doing to help me. I agreed to continue my classes and wait for the new computer.

I just couldn't allow myself to sit around and wait for others to do what I knew I could do for myself though. On Valentine's Day, I went to Walmart and bought myself a new computer. I also purchased Office and JAWS for it. I wasn't too upset about having to do this. I did a little research and found out how to accomplish all of this for a fraction of what I used to spend on a computer and accessibility. Once again, I was proud of myself because I took care of it on my own.

VR came through with the new computer in record time. This replacement computer really acted like a new computer. It works great! I'm using it right now as a matter of fact.

I learned a lot about my own power when I advocate for myself. Being in a place that is actually equipped to teach the blind has proven very beneficial as well.

Chapter 7

*D*uring all of the events I discussed in the last few chapters, I was continuing to live my life in many other ways as well. I was seeing Lancelot through all of this and growing stronger and more confident as time went by. He was treating me with all his various skills. As this was happening, I was very rapidly changing and growing with all the new and positive stimuli.

One day Lancelot talked to me about my job goal with voc rehab. He pointed out my schedule wouldn't be my own if I worked for someone else. I had always been at the beck and call of others . . . was this what I wanted for my future as well?

I looked at what I had learned since I moved to Mesa. I realized I had some pretty cool skills in my repertoire. I had begun my Reiki training. Lancelot talked me into getting my life coaching training as well. I knew very well the power I already possessed in my keen ability to communicate with others.

Combined with the unique skills and abilities God had already gifted me with, I realized who I had been becoming my entire life. I knew for certain what God had created me to do. I was shocked at how certain I was this was correct. I could literally see how every little pain that had been inflicted upon my entire being throughout my life had been preparing me for just this appointment. That's just what it felt like; a divine appointment. I had discovered my calling. I would become the world's most experienced life coach.

That conversation has certainly changed my life.

Today I'm not an administrative assistant. I'm an author, life coach and motivational speaker. I'm out in the world living my calling and finding fulfillment every single day. I can feel my being getting stronger constantly. If I had stuck with the administrative assistant racket, I would be stuck in one place and there would be very little room for me to continue to grow and learn. I feel strongly I should continue on this path now that I've stumbled upon it.

As I said earlier, I told Randi I wanted a divorce. I didn't feel free to do this when my mother-in-law was still living. It was more than four months after we lost mom before I was able to gather the courage to confront my husband.

The day I chose to do this I was physically ill. I was admitting I had failed at marriage; something I had never been allowed to do.

I was shocked when Randi's only concern was whether I'd been sleeping with my life coach. Of course, I hadn't. Once I told him this, he simply gave me up. He didn't want me unless he thought someone else might be in line. I realized my own husband didn't love me either. I had known it all along . . . a wife knows these things.

This helped me realize my decision to leave my husband was the correct one—even though everything I had ever been taught told me just the opposite. I decided if no one else loved me, I would have to figure out how to love myself. I felt very strongly I deserved to find true happiness after everything I had been through in Montana.

Randi and I went online and filled out divorce papers together. We were crying as we talked about everything we had been through together. I couldn't believe our marriage was ending like this. People tried to tear us apart for years with no luck. Now, here we were having beaten all of them, and yet we were still falling apart.

We printed the papers out. I took them down to the local courthouse here. I paid the filing fee and the divorce was filed.

As I was doing this, I kept asking myself, *"Was the end of my marriage one of the things those stupid doctors had predicted all those years ago? Had they guessed what I was truly capable of or was I right all along?" I knew only time would tell.*

The day Randi and our kids loaded up and left town was horrible. I stood at the end of my driveway all alone and waved with tears streaming down my face as my children left me. Was I making the right decision?

All I could do was cling to my faith in the spirit that had always guided me. I felt utterly alone as I turned and walked back into my large, newly empty house.

Today, over four years later, I'm still married to Randi. I'm finding that taking my life back has been a much larger undertaking than I surmised.

In the weeks after my family left, I found out to proceed with my divorce, I would have to locate and refile the identical forms I had already filled out. I thought at first, *no problem, I can solve this one of several ways.* I truly wasn't worried. I've become very adept at problem-solving over the last thirty years. Here is what happened . . .

First, I called my local courthouse and inquired about any services that might be available here for me to use—either free or paid, I wasn't concerned. I just needed a number I could call to make an appointment to go in and talk to someone about helping me do this.

I was utterly shocked when I was told there was no such service here. What did blind people do for legal aid here?

At this point, I didn't have time to pursue it further, so I was forced to let my divorce lapse.

I eventually met a blind man who turned me onto his attorney. The guy took a retainer from me and then told me he couldn't help me, I had to contact an attorney in Montana.

After losing all that money on that sleaze bag I gave up for a while. Randi and I had never been at each other's throats so maybe we could just let things ride as they were for a while.

Eventually, I met a deaf driver who turned me onto his attorney. This guy also promised to help me get my divorce refiled. He wouldn't return my calls after I gave him a large retainer.

By now I was getting really sick of attorneys and their bullshit. I'm still married today. I've given up on being able to live my life for myself.

Chapter 8

The month before I told Randi I wanted a divorce I visited my doctor for what should have been a fairly routine appointment. I nearly swallowed my tongue when the nurse converted the kilograms into pounds for me. I weighed in at a hefty 298 pounds.

I had never been so heavy in my life and it terrified me! This was the straw that broke the camel's back as they say.

I knew I had to take matters into my own hands. I couldn't allow myself to just get sicker and sicker and then eventually die from obesity. I had been through far too much to just let my life end like that. I knew what I had to do.

The very day after my family left, I woke up early and hit my treadmill.

I did a smart thing in putting my treadmill in my bedroom—right where it would be easily accessible to me first thing each morning. I think that was a big key to my success.

That first morning was rough. My entire being hurt.

I was careful not to put any unrealistic expectations on myself initially. I experienced many different "personal trainer" types in my time. The arbitrary guidelines that were always used just drove me crazy. Just who decided what was "normal?" For me, just being able to walk and talk again was a big accomplishment.

I realized long ago, if I was doing my very best—or if I were striving to make my performance better than the last time I performed the task in question—this meant I was improving, even if no one else saw it with *their* measuring stick.

Basically, I decided to always compete against myself in life. If I could do better than myself, then nothing else mattered. I knew I didn't have a prayer if I tried to compete at the same level as my sighted peers who hadn't suffered the same unique set of physical challenges I had overcome.

This is the same philosophy I employed when I worked out. I pushed myself to perform a bit harder each morning. My strategy worked. It wasn't long before I found my body literally running to get on the treadmill each morning. I had to hold myself back; my body craved the exercise so much. I found I had a ready supply of energy throughout each day as well. It was great!

I remember watching my children playing with their friends when they were younger. I wondered if I ever had that much energy. I couldn't think of such a time. I had been so sick as a child. I wondered back then if there was a way to flip this mysterious switch back in the opposite direction so an adult could once again have this level of energy.

If so, could *I* find that switch? I feared I may be reaching for something as elusive as the legendary fountain of youth.

I committed myself to my early morning workout routine. I experienced results almost immediately. Each morning I felt a little better than the day before. I was experiencing greater levels of energy each day as well. It became so intense I couldn't sit down. It was like I had ADHD. Now that I had so much energy, it was easy to find things to do. I increased my workout time each morning. I was constantly moving and feeling great.

I found many techniques to help me in my journey to better health.

I knew I would need my own gage to measure my progress if this was going to work. I needed to know on a regular basis if I were losing weight and if so, how much? I couldn't read my bathroom scale. I went and found a talking scale and then I was able to track my progress.

I began weighing on the same day and time each week so I would have a measure that would be as accurate as possible.

Over time, I have experienced a great deal of success from working out.

One day I went on Facebook and posted my results from weighing that morning. I received a lot of praise from my friends. I thrived on the words of encouragement I was receiving each week. It became so bad I had to force myself to stop posting; I was becoming so vain.

Over time the grief of losing my family became too much for me to bear. I found I was overwhelmed with sadness and would burst into tears without provocation. I took a leave of absence from school to get myself in order.

I started seeing a shrink during this time. He was highly qualified and very expensive. I was concerned about my psychological health. I was angry, confused and very terrified. I wasn't certain what to expect from myself during this time. What else could I do?

I saw that guy for over a year. I started my life coaching training during this time.

I remember the day I realized I had to fire this doctor.

We were in session and he was "treating" me like every other doctor in his profession had always done.

As I was trying to talk to him, he kept walking right over the top of me. He was so busy telling me what his opinion was he wasn't even listening to his patient anymore!

What really occurred to me was I had been getting something much better from my life coach.

Once I was able to get my doctor's attention, I told him about my classes. I also told him about the last one I attended earlier that month. During that class, we discussed with each other how to determine a fair fee to charge our clients for our life coaching services. I informed him I figured I should charge at least what *he* was charging me because I had learned a better way. I didn't bother to tell him I wouldn't be back. I laughed all the way to the bank.

I was feeling very rebellious after I left my husband.

While out on leave, I went and qualified for my medical marijuana card. My husband was telling me for years I should get it when we lived in Montana. I had been suffering for an awfully long time at that point. I refused because I had small children at home back then. Once I no longer had that responsibility, I felt free to get my card.

I was instantly amazed at what I experienced. Not only did I have a great deal of pain relief, but the plant even took away most of my anxiety! I realized rather quickly how much my anxiety had been crippling me over the years once it was gone.

Over time I integrated various strategies into my life to aid in my recovery. I bought an echo dot for $50. That was the best grant I ever spent. Having access to unlimited music by just requesting it? I was in seventh heaven! I quickly connected my echo dot to a blue tooth soundbar in my bedroom so the soothing strains filled my entire master bedroom. I also utilized some of my favorite fragrances as a type of aromatherapy around my home.

I learned how to utilize meditation during my workouts. I became so comfortable meditating I was able to use it in my weight loss as well.

I had a large mirror attached to the wall in front of my treadmill. I Could sort of see my reflection in the glass. That was only a small part of my reason for wanting the mirror though. I was experiencing some interesting stuff with my vision due to my constant use of marijuana. Improving my vision hadn't been of much interest to me for many years though. I wanted to use the mirror more as a prop—something to signify what I was experiencing in my life, my changing perspective. How better to change your outlook than to do it by gazing into a looking glass?

The visual I always used when I did this was simple. I visualized millions of fat cells just sluffing off of my body as I walked all those miles on my treadmill. It was similar to the way dead skin cells are sluffed off without us even realizing it each and every day. I visualized my fat was disappearing the same way, and it happened just like that. I told myself I could and would literally walk out of my oversized, sick body and into the trim, sleek healthy one I imagined in the mirror. I kept that goal always in front of me when I was on my treadmill. My treadmill was where I took the first steps on this journey to find my healthier, trimmer self.

I imagined this weight was just slipping away the more I walked. I focused all my attention on thinking that.

Of course, I tried to manage this process with diet also. I have never been able to count calories for obvious reasons. I grew sick and tired of asking sighted people to help me calculate calorie or fat content for me just so I could diet. I had to figure out how to eat better without the same tools most people can use.

It probably wasn't the best way to go about it, but this is what I did to my body.

I stopped drinking all coffee products and soft drinks immediately. I also tried to eat less when I ate but I still ate whatever I wanted. I've never been very good about denying myself food because of how I was raised; we went hungry enough. If I ate a little more than I thought I should, I would simply work a little harder in my workout to take it off. This just gave my body even more of what it was craving so it was all good.

I also used Odwalla protein shakes and Carnation instant breakfast as meal replacements.

It wasn't long before people were literally exclaiming over how skinny I was becoming. I was dropping weight so fast. People who saw me every few days but not every day were always surprised at how much I had lost from one time to the next time when they would see me! This is what I was able to accomplish using my mind.

There was a time when I might have suspected people were just telling me what they thought I wanted to hear, but all my jeans were literally falling off of me during this time as well so I know how legit their words were. It was incredible!

I was also continuing to see Lancelot through all of this. The Reiki, yoga and massage therapy helped me on my path as well.

Chapter 9

*L*ancelot and I did many things together over time. Some of the sessions involved hypnotherapy. I was hypnotized on multiple occasions.

I think the one that impacted me the most was when he took me back to the early years of my blindness. I visualized my younger self; that little, terrified girl who I can still remember being.

In the vision, I spoke to and embraced my younger self. I did this as my older, more mature self.

The really eerie thing about it was this; all those years ago when I really *was* that terrified, little girl, I spent a lot of time gazing off into the distance on clear days. I was calling out to my future self, attempting to connect over the continuum—hoping to get some words of encouragement I could cling to during those dark years.

I am certain in my heart it was *my* own voice I was hearing back then. All those years ago I heard the voice of my future self echoing back to me over the decades, giving me the strength to carry on. I recognized it as soon as I heard it when Lancelot hypnotized me. So, what came first, the chicken or the egg?

Before I met Lancelot, it was only God who was certain I had a purpose. I only *suspected* it back then. Once I was able to hear my truth clearly as it was screamed at me from my very soul, I realized God had been whispering the truth in my ear all along. I suddenly knew I was right all those years. It really *didn't* matter what the doctors or anyone else had been saying, what *did* matter was I had known what the truth was all along. This is where I finally found my strength that set me free. This absolute certainty was very refreshing after so many years of fighting to prove it.

Breaking free from the need to meet others' approval really helped my self-esteem. I had been working on doing this for many years. When my life coach helped me finish the process, it was a really big deal for me. I became so good at my new way of thinking, I noticed rather quickly that other people, especially the opposite sex, started recognizing how intelligent and beautiful I was as well. It was crazy! I never had so many people fawning for my attention. These were people online as well as in every area of my life.

Chapter 10

When Randi and my children left, I was so scared I would have some kind of break down. I cried all the time in private. It was all I could do to make it to the ladies' room when at school before I would break down. Since my heart was so shattered, I just tried my best to suck it up and worked on healing my body and brain for a while.

As time went by, I began to develop friendships all over the place because I was participating in so many different activities. I was taking part in any new enterprise I could find in an effort to bring more diversity into my life. This strategy worked well in Missoula to help me with my growth, so I tried it again.

It has been a marvelous success!

It has felt similar to when I was overcoming my arrested childhood and the bull crap that came from that TBI. This process was interrupted when I was in my early twenties. Now, I finally had the opportunity to finish it. I believe I have been able to exercise most of that horrible phantom from my psyche at last. This has been a remarkable journey; one I'm going to try to recount for my readers.

I was continuing my Reiki training during this time as well as many other interesting pursuits.

I met a blind guy on a chat group, and we became nearly constant phone buddies.

Bernie was always having slumber parties with these two blind women who lived near him. I thought, *what a great idea; blind friends to hang out with.* This began my search for a blind friend who lived nearby to hang out with.

I was on one of my favorite Facebook groups for blind people one day and was chatting with someone who seemed pretty cool, so I took a peek at his profile. It said he lived in Phoenix.

Cool beans! I sent him a private message suggesting we exchange phone numbers.

One thing led to another and he was at my front door a few days later.

This began one of the most interesting relationships of my life.

My Big EQ became very special to me during the course of our relationship.

He is a totally blind artist. I stumbled upon him strictly by accident; or by the hand of God, take your pick.

When EQ lived with me, I experienced one of the best times of my life. I had a companion who didn't have sloppy habits. He was organized and put stuff away. I didn't have to deal with the frustrations I had always put up with while living with sighted people.

I had always believed my blind friends who chose to be with blind partners just felt they were not good enough for a sighted spouse. Now I was learning what a great experience it was.

I have to tell you, all facets of our relationship were made richer due to our mutual blindness. Not just how we both took each other's needs into consideration but the time we spent together was so meaningful. I was amazed at the levels of intimacy we were able to achieve.

Just any blind person would not have done though. EQ and I had a lot in common other than just our blindness. We are both independent thinkers and creators. He was the first blind person I've met who wasn't scared to go literally anywhere with his cane; like me. This was awesome. I finally had a companion who took on life at a similar speed to mine.

This was not only my first serious relationship with a blind man; it was also my first live-in relationship. I felt like I was becoming a "woman of the world."

I went to the NFB convention by myself again that summer. I invited EQ, but he couldn't come.

I was living a highly active, busy life at this point. It was three days before I left for the convention when it happened.

Chapter 11

*I*t was a Thursday afternoon when it happened. I was taking my trash out and stumbled on the edge of the curb because my hands were too full, and I wasn't using proper cane technique.

I actually had my cane tucked under my arm and was going to use it on the way back to the house, but it just didn't work out as planned.

When I fell, I landed very hard on my rear end. At first, I wasn't sure what to do; I was in shock. It was very painful, immediately.

I stumbled into the house. I wasn't sure I should even be walking, it hurt so bad.

First, bathroom to pee. Then into the kitchen to grab water from the refrigerator, and finally into the living room to collapse into my chair and figure out what to do.

Ouch! Fuck . . . I forgot already!

Once I pulled myself together enough to be somewhat presentable, I called a Lyft to the nearest urgent care facility.

After finally getting an x-ray I was informed I had busted my ass. There was nothing they could do except give me some pain meds and send me home.

I frantically explained to the doctor I was supposed to leave for Florida in three days. I sought his counsel.

I established with him there was nothing they could do for me. He agreed if I had trouble with my tail bone while I was in Florida, I would be able to go to the emergency room there as easily as I would be able to do if I stayed home and felt sorry for myself.

It didn't take me long to decide I was not going to let my busted tail bone prevent me from enjoying this convention. So, I went.

I spent the three days leading up to my departure doing everything I could think of to get ready. I went and purchased an inflatable ring I could sit on when I was forced to sit down on my trip. I worked hard to keep moving while my muscles were trying to seize up on me. It was very painful walking those first few days, but I knew I couldn't stop.

I also worked diligently to get off of the hard stuff my doctor gave me for pain relief. I opted to take my medical marijuana with me for pain management while I was gone.

It turned out to be an amazing trip all things considered.

I was able to participate in a fair amount of the convention activities. I remember walking to and from as many of the seminars as I was able to manage with my injury. I also made new friends who I hung out with in their rooms or mine that week. I not only made it to at least part of the banquet on the final night but I even had a hook-up that week.

The most important thing this experience taught me was I can do a lot even when I'm in severe pain. Of course, my medical marijuana helped along the way.

As I write this passage, it has been over two years since I broke my tail bone. Breaking my tail bone has greatly complicated my health.

Chapter 12

*L*ife with EQ continued undaunted for months. Over that summer we began spending a lot of time together. He gradually moved into my home.

In October of that year, Bernie flew out for a visit and stayed with EQ and me. We shared some good times together when Bernie was here. As I said, I was realizing how awesome it was to have blind friends to hang out with.

How I wish my parents hadn't forbidden me from engaging with the blind community as a child. My life as a teenager was such a lonely existence.

Life went on fairly smoothly for weeks, even months. All this time I was continuing to rebuild my body in spite of my tail bone. I just concentrated on working even harder to strengthen my gluteus muscles.

Life was great. EQ and I were so compatible. I just knew it was doomed to end; I could feel it in my heart. I always knew I wasn't supposed to be so happy.

EQ kept his rental even though he was spending most of his time at my house. It turned out to be a good thing. During this time EQ's roommate from his other place began hanging out at my house also.

At first, having Paul here wasn't a problem at all. He cooked for EQ and me and stayed out of our hair for the most part.

That December one of my sons decided to move in with us.

Wayne asked for a dog right away. Our family dog went back to Montana with Randi.

Buddy was eventually killed in our front yard. A crazy female deer who was giving birth to a couple of fawns in the neighbor's yard jumped our fence and kicked the crap out of our blind old dog, right there in town! The deer population in Missoula was really getting out of hand.

I liked the idea of us getting a dog so I set about figuring out how to make it happen. Wayne and I both had school every day so no one would be home to let the dog out.

At the time I had a married couple cleaning the house for me. The husband was really good at problem-solving so I knew he was the one I should talk to.

Enlisting Bert's help turned out to be a good idea. He did all the research about how to install a reliable dog door in my house. After he presented the plan to me, I authorized him to proceed and we had our dog door shortly thereafter. Next came the dog.

My son went online and found a great dog on the Humane Society's website. We went and picked the dog up on Good Friday that spring. She was our Easter gift from God as far as I could tell. At least I hoped God was involved.

The lady at the Humane Society didn't introduce the dog to me at the shelter. She allowed my son to take over the adoption process. Because of this I eventually wound up with a sick, cranky dog in my house whom I couldn't see and who was a threat to my safety. Just imagine it!

We took the dog home that day.

After about a week I received a phone call from the Humane Society informing me my dog may have been exposed to "Valley Fever." This is a condition that is common here in Arizona. My understanding is it is in the soil and cannot be avoided. We all breathe in the spores every day. I've known humans who've contracted it. This was my first canine case of it though.

I loved Princess Leia by this time and was not going to reject her because of this.

Treating a dog for valley fever is a very expensive, time-consuming process. I have been treating her for over two years now. Her mood and behavior have definitely changed but they're still telling me she has it, so I still buy the expensive medicine.

I made a commitment to this animal when I adopted her. She has more than earned her keep in my life. She is remarkable. I will be talking more about her.

Chapter 13

My son was a pot smoker before he moved in with me. Having access to my medical marijuana only made a bad situation worse.

I knew if I chased him around and badgered him about it, I would be fighting a losing battle. Imagine how this would have gone?

I certainly wasn't going to spend my son's entire time here alienating him like many parents do. I knew I was even more helpless when it came to monitoring his behavior when he was away from me than most parents are. I wasn't about to enter that fight. It was only pot after all. This was how I reasoned it out anyway.

It wasn't long before my son wouldn't get out of bed to go to school. He loved school when he was young. As he grew older it became more about his friends than his homework, but he still went.

When Wayne became wrapped up in pot, he just lost all interest in being happy and having friends.

He began sitting around whining about how bad he had it. He was using all the familiar victimhood phrases about being lonely, misunderstood and all that stuff—the things we all feel when we are teenagers.

He also used his father and my separation as just another excuse for his bad behavior. I wasn't having any of it!

Believe me, I had him beaten hands down in the department of who had the worse struggle as an adolescent; he wasn't getting any sympathy from his mother.

I was really concerned about how weak my son had become. How would he ever survive in the real world?

My son had lived here for about a month when something really strange happened.

It actually started the night before. We had a party here at our house that night.

We had blind guests at the party as well as sighted guests.

There were people here from several different walks of life; I try to keep my life very diverse.

We had music playing and there were guests all over the house and back yard. These were all people I knew.

There were no disturbances during the party, just people laughing and visiting. My friends all knew I only invited people I trusted to my home.

EQ and I were the host and hostess of the party that night. Everything went well.

It was the next morning when all hell broke loose . . .

Chapter 14

 awoke to the sound of my son yelling. He was addressing EQ. He said something like, "Get the F*** out of my face, man!"

His voice was coming from the other side of my closed bedroom door. I couldn't get a clear idea of what was going on if I remained in my room. I rushed out into the main living area where my son and EQ were still engaged in a heated argument.

I was totally baffled.

I learned my son was asleep on the couch. He opened his eyes to find my blind boyfriend "glaring" down at him. My son was understandably upset.

I was perplexed. How do you explain to a teenaged boy a totally blind person really can't glare? As someone who has been both sighted and blind, I must say it is my belief many facial expressions are learned from seeing them.

I actually have proof of this. As a mother, I can't count the number of times I've spoken to other parents. Our conversations often focused on our children. The hilarious tales about over-exaggerated facial expressions our children have exhibited in their organic interaction with each other . . .

Their expressions are exaggerated because they are learning to form them for the first time; they don't come naturally like a smile might.

Therefore, if a person has never had the opportunity to learn to glare in anger, why would they do this?

I think there is a good chance EQ's eyes looked like he was glaring because he was squinting in concentration. It's completely plausible he brushed up against my son's face when he bent to check out the sounds he was hearing. In the process, he woke my son up, startling him.

I have literally had identical experiences myself many times over the years. Whatever was going on, I don't believe EQ was glaring, not consciously anyway. I think the whole situation may have started with a simple misunderstanding that snowballed way out of control.

Anyway, when Wayne opened his eyes, he felt threatened by EQ's proximity to him. I suspect EQ may have bent down to listen to him while he slept or to identify a sound he heard. He may not have even known my son was laying there asleep if he didn't happen to touch him.

I have literally had the same experience more than once over the years—that is, surprising a sleeping person who is laying somewhere unusual.

When Wayne opened his eyes, he flipped out, like many people might do in similar circumstances.

I think this all happened nearly simultaneously and just before I walked onto the scene. When I interrupted the situation, it seemed to confuse things a bit more.

I was able to get them to stop yelling at each other. Wayne went out to the front yard to cool off. EQ and I went into my bedroom.

I was sitting on the edge of my bed a few minutes later when I heard a strange noise coming from the front of my home. EQ was at the foot of the bed and I was sitting on the edge of the bed facing the doorway where the noise was coming from.

My first thought was, *Hmmm, there's a parade out front? Well, it's Saturday after all!*

Then I realized the chanting noise sounded very angry. My next thought was, *riot?*

None of this made much sense but at that moment, nothing made sense.

It felt like my life was caught up in some kind of gigantic, energetic vortex . . . My life had been controlled by this power before.

That day I felt this mighty hand influencing the situation in a huge way. I knew I better proceed with caution.

I took a couple of steps towards the front entryway of my home, listening to the bizarre sounds coming from outside. It sounded like there were a lot of angry people marching out there, it was very strange.

Suddenly my front door flew open. My son charged through it. I struggled to see who all the other people were whom I had heard outside. I never saw anyone else.

As my son charged towards me, I could hear him babbling in a loud, unintelligible voice. Some of the words seemed kind of clear but then other words would come out of his mouth that sounded all twisted up—like there was more than one person trying to talk at the same time. It definitely didn't sound or feel like it was my own son right here in front of me speaking that day. It reminded me of how it felt to listen to a person delivering a message in tongues in church.

This was all happening simultaneously; it was a lot for my brain and psyche to absorb.

My son charged further into the house. I retreated back into my bedroom.

As I turned to face my advancing son, I was suddenly impressed with an image of him reaching out to strangle me with his bare hands. This did not happen.

When I saw this image, I reached out towards my advancing son. I slid my right hand up the back of his neck, threading my fingers through his hair. I tightened my grip on his hair, arresting his advance upon me. This all happened in a split second.

I was immediately struck with the impression something unorthodox was going on. I knew instinctively conventional reactions may not be the best. I instantly released my hold on his hair. I let my hand gently pat his shoulder as it fell away.

It was too late. My son was reacting defensively. His fist shot out and socked me right in the eye.

Chapter 15

*M*y world stood still. I wasn't quite sure what was happening for a few moments. Then I cried out, "Someone call 911, my son just punched me in the face!"

I said this to warn EQ wherever he was my son was not right. I wanted to make sure no one else wound up hurt. I wasn't the only blind person in the house at this point.

I shrunk from the words I had just uttered. How could my son have punched his blind mother in the face? It was wrong on so many levels. It still makes no sense today, over two years later.

I was immediately struck by several things in that moment of clarity.

First, my son hit me in the right eye. This is my dominant eye. It is also the same eye my own mother punched me in when I was a teenaged girl myself. Talk about generational curses!

I felt so exposed.

My family had gone through so much when I was a kid . . . were my children doomed to repeat the cycle of abuse? How was I going to stop the nightmare from repeating itself?

I now knew what the common denominator was; it was me. If I removed myself from the equation, would it save my children?

It's been a long, arduous journey since that fateful morning over two years ago.

That day I had to go to the urgent care to get looked at. As I was leaving in my Lift, Potter, another of my blind friends who stayed the night was making contact with his ride as well. I was in severe pain and very, very concerned about my neurological health. I barely noted Potter's departure as I fled for the urgent care.

The staff at the urgent care know me because I've been there on my own behalf or with various friends or family over time. The first thing the lady said to me when she saw my shiner was, "We can't see you here honey, you need to get that x-rayed at the emergency room."

I think she realized I was about to fall to pieces, I was barely holding it together at that point. She helped direct me to the emergency room.

At the ER I was checked in. I had to get an x-ray of my face to make sure my eye socket wasn't broken. The way I felt, I thought it was a good idea.

I insisted I had no interest in speaking to a police officer. I had no intention of pressing charges against my own son. Like I have been saying all along, something strange was going on.

To my horror, my thoughts and wishes did not matter.

I found out that day here in Arizona there is a zero-tolerance policy when it comes to domestic violence.

The state will pursue justice on the victim's behalf.

The officers ignored my attempts to reason with them as they left the ER on their way to my home to talk to my son that day. The last thing I yelled at them as they were leaving the hospital was something like, "I know my rights and I forbid you now from speaking to my son without me present!" (I was pretty sure this was correct and even if it wasn't, I had learned from previous experience that police officers rarely know what our rights truly are.)

This is why they trample on them all the time. Scary . . . isn't it?

I'm telling you right now,—this is probably the most important lesson of my entire story, both parts—**learn your rights in order to protect them or they will be taken from you!** It happened to me. I know there are people lurking in our government right now who want to take away the rights of all Americans, not just me. We better wake up before it's too late!

That day I was trying desperately to keep something even more dreadful from happening before I could get back to my house. I knew what a hot head my son could be when he let his mouth run out of control.

He had voiced the typical anti-law enforcement rhetoric in the past I had been hearing from people for years. I was absolutely terrified my son would engage with the officers before I could get home.

Once I was done at the ER, I debated if I should go straight home or stop by the pharmacy to get my prescription filled first.

I realized once I went home, I'd probably be busy all night getting this crazy situation straightened out. I stopped at the pharmacy en route.

When I finally arrived at my home, I found my son standing out in front of our house chatting with the police officers who had come to the hospital.

I really had no idea what was going to happen during this time. It was so scary.

The officers swore us both to tell the truth. Then they asked us what had happened.

Our stories lined up; he had hit me in the right eye.

That was all the officers needed to hear. They both took a step towards my son saying at the very same moment, "Please put your hands behind your back."

I was in shock. I was watching my son being arrested in front of my very eyes. Imagine that? I was absolutely terrified.

I jumped to attention immediately. I demanded to know from the officers exactly where they were taking my son and how I could gain access to him. I had never been to a police station and had no idea how to find the one here in Mesa. What if I lost my son, literally?

The officers actually refused to give me any real information! I was shocked. How could they just come into my house and take my child away without having to tell me where they were taking him?

All they would tell me was I should sit and wait for a phone call that would come through. They promised the caller would give me directions on where and how I could go get my son.

Then I watched them march my eldest son out of my house to their waiting squad car in the street. I still don't know how I kept from losing it right there.

Chapter 16

The phone call came just as the officers promised. I was choking with relief as I answered the call. A very kind lady spoke gently to me and answered all my questions. She was patient with me while I found my device to record the info so I wouldn't forget it as soon as I hung up the phone.

When I arrived at the facility to "bail" my son out, I knew what it was to feel ashamed. People's reactions when they saw me, a blind woman with a big black eye approaching them, it was shocking.

This made me angry. Why should I feel ashamed? I had done nothing wrong.

I decided I would wear my shiner with pride—it was a battle scar earned through intense misery as far as I was concerned.

My entire life had been full of similar painful experiences.

Like I've said before, we can't grow and become better, stronger people if we don't face these sorts of difficult experiences in life.

I've become a firm believer in the saying, "What doesn't kill you will make you stronger." Difficulties in life are just part of the natural development process. The more difficult the challenge, the greater the potential for growth. The key is learning to recognize these huge potentials for growth and knowing how to harness them, so you get the full benefit.

I took my son back home with me. There was no one else here when we finally arrived. EQ and Paul had cleared out after the officers had left with my son in cuffs earlier that day.

It was surreal; coming back into the house where it all began. It had started like any other day but had gone off the rails somehow. What would be next in our lives?

I was half terrified, half excited. I knew there were bound to be big things in both our futures now. The very power of God had been released into both our lives, that was what I felt that day. We just had to steer it in the right direction.

Chapter 17

T hose early days were interesting, to say the least. I found myself experiencing flashbacks to the events of that Saturday morning. Something as simple as my son suddenly appearing behind me from nowhere would send me into a screaming, tear-filled flashback. Any sudden noises had similar effects on me . . . I was a real mess.

I took a picture of my face and texted it to my son's father in Montana. It was a horrific photo to behold.

Returning to school meant exposing my black eye to the world. Thank God I went to a blind school where most of the people had some level of vision loss.

I was reeling for a long time after my son assaulted me.

I posted the story of what had happened on Facebook.

My "friends" and family all over the place were up in arms about what happened. I was advised by several of them I should send my son away.

I struggled with this concept. What good would that do? His father was in much worse health than I was.

I knew intellectually I wasn't in true danger from my son.

My son wasn't even angry at me that day. It was him and EQ who had experienced the disagreement.

I knew that day and I believe to this day the entire situation was beyond Wayne's and my control. There was another force making events happen that day.

Regardless of how or why it happened, we had to move on somehow.

Those early weeks were interesting. My heart and mind were in a tailspin. Imagine everything I had coursing through my psyche?

Spending time alone with Wayne after what happened was surreal. As anyone would expect, we talked over what had happened.

We agreed we did not mean each other any harm that day.

When reflecting back on the events that occurred at the party the night before the assault, a strange possibility rose to my consciousness.

Wayne was describing some very peculiar behavior from one of the guests at the party that night.

He described this guest walking from room to room in our house throughout the evening. This guy had some kind of talisman in his hand he was stroking while he was doing this.

During this time, this guy could be heard mumbling under his breath.

I recalled seeing that freak behaving in just that strange manner myself. I saw that blind guy in every single room of my house that night, including my walk-in closet.

Sounds bizarre, doesn't it?

The night of the party I was too distracted waiting on guests to give it much thought.

I assumed this "friend" could be trusted just because he was blind. I of all people should have known better than to underestimate a fellow blind person.

This wasn't my first interaction with this individual. I had invited this same creepy guy out to other social gatherings previously. It had been my goal to help him develop better social skills so he would feel more comfortable in social gatherings.

At many of those events, I had overheard other friends commenting on similar strange behavior from him. I even witnessed it firsthand when a girlfriend made a point of bringing it to my attention at trivia one night. I remember how eerie it was listening to him that night.

After looking at the history of strange behavior from this individual an eerie possibility rose to my mind.

I had learned about spiritual warfare from Marjory all those years ago in Missoula. This situation had all the earmarks she had taught me to look for.

(See author's previous work *Because You're Blind*.) I now knew how I needed to look at this situation in order to overcome it; I was at war.

Chapter 18

As time went by Wayne continued to refuse to go to school or be obedient to me in any way. It was ridiculous. I couldn't enforce any rules over my son for fear he might blow up on me. I finally sent him back to his father in Montana.

Looking back, I should have realized the day he punched me we would eventually come to that point. I kept my son here with me as long as I could.

On Good Friday that spring Wayne and I went to the Humane Society and picked up Princess Leia.

I found it significant she came with the name of a magical princess.

The fact we met her on Good Friday, a day we recognize God's blessings, only made my faith stronger.

We brought Princess home that day.

My son immediately informed me she was his dog and I was to stay away from her. I laughed inside. I knew she was my dog from day one. My son was a typical kid—he didn't want the responsibility of a dog.

I, on the other hand, had always secretly wanted a dog of my very own.

Princess has played a significant role in my life since we brought her home that spring day.

In the beginning, she slept in Wayne's room. She would growl at me in a low voice each time I stuck my head in his doorway to greet her. She had some real social issues in those early days.

One day I caught Wayne speaking cruelly to Princess. When I heard his loud, intentionally harsh words directed at an innocent creature, I was reminded of all the times in my life when other people had treated me in a similar fashion. I was reminded of thirty years of pain from similar abusive treatment. This was the guy who had punched me in the face a few months before. Imagine how I was feeling at that point? It was then I called his father to discuss options.

His dad suggested Wayne could submit to a "voluntary" psychological examination that would last three days. After this time, assuming Wayne passed, he would return to my home.

My son refused.

This put me in a tough spot. I had to be concerned for my safety.

That Sunday I put my son on the plane back to his father in Montana.

Chapter 19

When Wayne departed for Montana, he left a bad situation in his wake in the form of his dog. I had no relationship with Princess at that point. Wayne had been keeping her isolated in his bedroom. I knew she had been having some accidents in there over time. I had to get her out of there and get his room cleaned up. This was easier said than done.

Each time I tried to get up the courage to go into his room, Princess would growl at me from somewhere within the shadowy confines of my son's bedroom. This would scare me, and I'd run away again. It was silly.

I called my housekeeper. She laughed at me when I told her about my predicament. She came over to give me a hand with my big, scary princess.

She helped me put a leash on Princess so we could take her outside. As soon as I got her outside and took the leash off her collar she ran right back in the house and hid in my son's room again.

This time I not only shut my son's bedroom door but I shut the outside door so she couldn't come back in the house right away. I hung out in the backyard with her for a while.

Then I opened the door so she could come in the house if she chose to. She decided she preferred life outside by the pool.

She spent the next several weeks out in the back yard. She acted like she was on some kind of retreat at a luxurious spa somewhere; it was funny.

I checked on her first thing each morning. A stop at the back door to check on her each afternoon when I returned from class became routine.

I would even go out there in the middle of the night to speak to her and check on her. She always made noises, so I knew she was okay during those visits.

I put out fresh water and food for her during those days. She was just living in the backyard. The weather was absolutely breathtaking so who could blame her? She was doing a lot of healing during that time and I gave her the space to do it.

One day that summer it was very hot outside. I realized I had to get Princess in the house so she would be safe.

At first, she wouldn't budge from her spot by the pool. It took a lot of prodding from my housekeeper and me to get her back in the house.

As soon as she was back inside, she found her new sanctuary. It turned out my walk-in closet located in my master suite made a great castle for a princess.

The first morning after Princess moved into my closet, I started my dog campaign.

I had been wanting to get out and walk for exercise for a while, but I had no one to walk with. Having a dog in my closet gave me a splendid idea.

Princess became my new walking buddy. We started small. I would set the timer on my device for ten minutes and we'd start to make our way around our block. When the timer went off, we'd turn around and start back home. We did this for a while increasing our time each morning.

The first morning I clicked the leash on Princess's collar, I had to gently tug to get her to her feet. The second morning she came along a little more willingly. By the third or fourth day, she was leaping to her feet and running for the front door. At that point, I knew my Princess was now my dog for sure.

I tried to make it a habit to take her out each time I returned home. Princess started meeting me at the front door when I got home from class each afternoon, wagging her tail in anticipation of our afternoon walk. We developed a rigorous walking schedule.

While out on our walk one day we came to an intersection. As we stepped up onto the curb, I could feel the wind as the cars were zooming past us. We were no longer on our quiet, secluded, cul-de-sac.

Princess and I both hesitated for a moment. I could feel her pressing back against my legs in fear. She didn't want to continue along the sidewalk where the cars were speeding past.

She reminded me of myself the past few years. I had been finding a lot of opportunities to step out and take chances in life.

At first, I had played it safe, taking no chances.

Then I realized I wasn't living my life.

When I got out of court in January of 2012 with my constitutional rights intact, I was so angry I had lost fifteen years of self-determination. I wanted to make the rest of my life really count for something.

I realized back then I had to stop "standing outside the fire" if I were going to make my mark on this world with the short time I have left here.

To me, this meant following my dreams and my heart, while trusting in my own good judgment. I had always been told my judgment was faulty . . . could I trust it now?

Well, I have trusted myself for a while now. What an exciting and interesting ride this has been! I can't believe what I've learned and accomplished in these last few years while I've been in charge of my own life.

I published my first book *"Because You're Blind"* in 2013. I left my husband in 2016. I founded my company, *Blue Butterfly Enterprises* in August of 2019. I then launched my YouTube channel, *Becca's World* in October of 2019. I hit 1,000 subscribers just before the first of the year. We're making a movie based on my first book at present and I'm writing my second book as we speak; literally.

I dare say, I have been doing a lot since I dissolved the guardianship. I could do nothing while under the guardianship. How can you make any plans when you have to get permission to do everything? It was so very frustrating. Just imagine it for a moment. It was quite literally my four parents and the state of Montana that were holding me back from achieving anything in life.

Chapter 20

My relationship with Princess definitely evolved over time. When we first brought her home, she was unfriendly and ill-tempered. Once she moved into my closet, I continued to give her space. I had my bed and she slept in the closet—period. Or so I thought.

One night Princess climbed right up on my comfy king-size bed and laid down beside me! Just imagine it . . .

She's like a big old ox. It's a good thing I have a large bed. She took up half of it herself. My mouth fell open as I gasped in shock.

I had been showing Princess with every word and deed since the day I brought her home I was truly devoted to her. Now, she was finally reaching back for companionship. It was remarkable.

This began a gradual process. Over time, Princess has come further out of her shell. She comes to me for affection. Today, she literally skips through my home with a smile on her face and her tail vigorously wagging. It's heart-warming to behold.

There were several key points in Princess's recovery. It has been so much fun to watch as she blossomed with more confidence each day. (She reminds me of myself.)

There were many changes in our lives over time. Some of the incidents that occurred have faded into the background. I'm going to discuss some of the more profound things I've experienced the last few years.

My life has felt like I've stumbled into the Twilight Zone many times—it's been so bizarre. I have no idea what a "normal" person's life is like. Maybe all people have the crazy things happen to them like what's been happening to me? All I know is my life is no longer the boring, stagnant existence it once was.

I guess it started when I followed through on my decision to leave Randi. I believe I shifted something just right in the matrix when I made that move. It was like I unleashed some kind of energy that has propelled me onward ever since.

Along with this energy, I have experienced a great deal of success in my endeavors. It feels like the results of my efforts are magnified. I feel like I have the favor of God Himself smiling down upon me. I believe I am receiving this favor because of my faithfulness all these years.

I took God at His word. The doctors said there was no hope for my recovery . . . what else could I do? I challenged God to come through on His promises, and He has. It's the most remarkable thing I've ever experienced. I am literally joyful every day as I watch the fulfillment of all His promises in my daily life.

How did I do this? It was a matter of changing my thinking so I was looking at my situation from a position of power and authority rather than one full of hopelessness and dependency.

When I saw my life from an eternal perspective—from God's point of view—I came to realize several important truths that have helped me overcome my situation. I'm going to try to explain them as well as I can in this book.

The first "truth" that has gotten me through is the following:

When you realize you were created by God and your only hope is to put what He said to the test, that faith can become the strength that leads you to your healing.

This is what I came to that spring day in 1989 when I initially woke up.

Ultimately, I figured out how to harness my belief in that Biblical creed until it became the fuel that has enabled me to manifest God's promises in my daily life.

It was only after I accepted my humanity that I received these promised blessings.

It started around the time I took up the cane.

Taking up the cane is a perfect metaphor for what I did.

Taking up the cane—and embracing who God had created me to be—became the beginning of my healing.

Chapter 21

Over time, after Wayne punched me, I became aware of a strong sense my life may be in danger. At first, it was just a feeling. Then I started noticing strange stuff. I began experiencing little "accidents" around my home. It was really strange.

I'd step down into my sunken bedroom only to have my foot roll out from under me because someone had placed a Styrofoam roller right up against the step down. I'd find other trip hazards conveniently set up in similar fashions around my living environment. It was unsettling, to say the least.

Then one morning as I was stepping into the shower, I slipped.

You might jump to the conclusion I had a misstep because of my vision. This was not what happened.

As I stepped onto the mat on the floor of my shower, it shot across the expanse of my shower stall. My legs went out from under me and I nearly bit the dust.

I strained my back and neck in my gyrations to stop my slide.

This was frightening enough but something even more terrifying happened in that same instant.

As I was struggling to regain my balance, I was struck with a case of déjà vu.

I had experienced nearly the same thing seven days before, the day after my housekeepers had done their regular weekly cleaning in my private bathroom.

When I realized this, my blood ran cold. What was going on? Just who could I trust?

It was at that point I started taking my feelings of being in danger a lot more seriously. I started "looking over my shoulder."

When I did a mental inventory of everyone I knew in Arizona, I realized to my horror there wasn't a single human being who I could turn to for protection. This left my dog as my only port in this developing storm.

I had allowed EQ and Paul to come back into my home. They proved more of a liability than an asset. With everything I was juggling at that point, I eventually realized I had to throw them both out for my own safety. I had to eliminate how many people had access to my private world.

I learned so many great things from this experience; mostly what I'm capable of when I stand up for myself. It was a fabulous growing experience.

The situation developed over time. It came to a head early one morning. I remember thinking how weird it was I kept having these significant events happen to me first thing in the morning. I guess it's because I always do my best thinking early when my mind and heart are fresh. Here's what happened.

I was peacefully walking through my house, opening my home up to welcome the new day. When I came across Paul, I greeted him with a hearty "Good morning!"

He chose that moment to blow up at me in return. He had actually been becoming more verbally confrontational over time.

That morning Paul snapped my last nerve. I had been more than accommodating to him and EQ for months with nothing but a headache for my efforts. I was getting sick of their mutually abusive treatment in return. I didn't need a couple of grown men who wanted to be taken care of. I had my own problems that needed attention.

Let me tell you, I have the gift of long-suffering. I put up with a lot of shit before I've had enough. Paul's the only man who has ever pushed me past that point.

That day I had experienced 'about enough' of his crap, it was time to cut the apron strings and put them both out to pasture. They were grown men who could fend for themselves. I was done playing mommy to a couple of overgrown babies.

Paul was easy to provoke. As I said all I had to do was greet him. So, I did.

He yelled at me in reply, just what I had come to expect from him.

I became good at swallowing my pain when I was forced to be around people who treated me rudely in Montana. I had made the conscious decision to leave that world behind. Why was I tolerating this abuse from the likes of Paul? He definitely wasn't worth the trouble.

I knew what needed to be done. So, I yelled back. Honestly, neither of us really sounded angry, just loud and stupid. It really felt scripted.

We did this for a few minutes.

I finally said, *"Get out if you don't like it. This is my house!"*

He grumbled around a lot, banging closet doors and slamming dresser drawers before storming out the front door. I'm sure he was hoping to wake EQ up to come to his aid. They had been ganging up against me for months.

I realized I had to divide them if I were going to conquer them.

Once Paul was gone, I went and woke EQ up.

EQ was sleepy and sweet at first. Then he commented he had overheard Paul and me yelling at each other.

I replied yes, we had a disagreement.

EQ took that opportunity to accuse me of being unreasonable to live with.

I had been hearing this ridiculous argument from him and Paul every time I asserted my wishes in my own house. I finally figured out how to win this one as well. Watch this.

Each time EQ complained about living in my house, I simply replied, "If you're unhappy here, maybe you should just leave."

It was the most obvious solution to his problem; there was just no way he could argue with my reasoning.

As my agreeing with him became my insistence that if he really felt this way, he should consider just moving out, the poor guy just gave up.

I made his happiness his own responsibility, not mine. This took away his ability to manipulate me. This has been a valuable lesson that has served me well ever since.

EQ was quickly growing frustrated with this new Becca. He liked the girl who idolized him and sought his approval. I had finally learned whose approval really mattered.

EQ quickly found his own way to the door that day. It was hard watching him go. We had been good together at one time.

I was thrilled I had finally woken up to reality. I just wish EQ had been so mature.

It wasn't very many days later when I received a message from another of my blind friends alerting me to EQ's activities on social media.

The immature little worm was spreading vicious lies about me on a local chat group specifically geared towards the blind community.

I shuddered as I listened to his vicious words when I finally had a chance to hear them. They were petty and lude—an obvious attempt to smear my reputation. I had no idea how far-reaching his words would be.

For a long time afterward—often when I would meet a new friend at a blind function—he or she would announce they had heard of me. Their reactions made it clear they had not liked the rumors.

The whole experience served to isolate me from the blind community. I was the "new kid" in town. EQ had spent much of his life here. I wound up the exiled stranger.

You can't keep a good dog down though. I wound up so much stronger in the end.

This experience worked to seal in my newfound self-confidence in a huge way. Believe me, my current boyfriend—the only guy I've been serious about since the day I threw EQ out—is totally put off at my ability to tell him he can take a hike if he's not happy. I have simply decided other people are responsible for their own happiness.

Chapter 22

hrowing Paul and EQ out didn't fix my problems, it only decreased them. I still felt very unsafe. It was horrible.

One day I took a dip in my pool. I was having a nice relaxing time.

As I swam around, I was abruptly seized with a strong feeling that I was being observed. I craned my head to look around me. I couldn't see anything at all.

It suddenly dawned on me how vulnerable I truly was. What would prevent someone from just climbing over the wall to finish me off?

I was hyperventilating a few minutes later as I frantically scrambled out of my pool.

Once I was safely back in the house, I kicked myself for my carelessness. I sat down and did an inventory of my daily activities. Just where were my vulnerable points?

I already knew my shower was dangerous. My most recent experience in there had confirmed this for me. I believed as long as I could keep my feet under me, I would have a fighter's chance for survival. This meant no more swimming.

I had to take care of my personal hygiene though. How was I supposed to make my shower safe?

Now, let me tell you, I've developed an interesting sense of humor as I've lived in this life. The following was literally the best solution I could come to at that point. I didn't do this to be funny.

I sought assistance from Bert for the job.

He had been my handyman anyway . . . what else was I supposed to do? I needed some stuff constructed for my safety.

I already had a few ideas in mind. It was simply a matter of implementing them.

In my first plan, I had Bert and his wife lay down strips on the floor of my shower. They were strips of rough material similar to what they put down in public pools to prevent slipping in the locker rooms.

Under my instruction and supervision, Bert and his wife painstakingly cut the material into strips that were a few inches long. Then after cleansing my shower floor, I had them secure them to the floor of my shower in strategic locations using an appropriate adhesive.

The whole process took several hours. I paid them both for their time just to try to make my shower safe for me to use.

Those strips only lasted a few days. It wasn't long before they were peeling up. It looked and felt terrible to step on. Back to the drawing board.

My next plan worked much better.

Again I engaged Bert's assistance. After purchasing two metal bars that were of appropriate length and strength, I directed Bert on exactly how and where to mount them in my shower. I told him to install a vertical bar just inside my shower door and a horizontal bar on the wall kitty-corner from that first bar.

I instructed him to use a stud finder to locate the studs inside the wall so the bars would be properly anchored to a strong support.

As I was doing this, I thought back to one particular day so many years ago when I was a newly blind, helpless teenager. I had the opportunity to learn from my stepfather that day. I spent time quizzing him on the proper use of a stud finder. Back then, I figured I would find that information helpful someday. I had no idea just how important the early teachings from my family and community would become.

Once Bert was done it was time for me to check on his handy work. Just how stable were these new bars? I wanted to make sure he had followed my instructions to the letter.

I stepped into my shower stall. I gripped both bars together and individually. I swung from them. I hung all my weight from them. They both stood up to the Becca Factor.

I knew I was good to go. If I slipped again, I would be able to grab either bar to catch myself.

Before this, I only slid across the floor out of control coming dangerously close to crashing through my glass shower walls. It had been so terrifying.

I was doing all of this stuff and changing my thinking to fit my new situation. I could feel it was time to press in and listen closely to that voice that had always guided me. It was a very cool experience.

Through all of this, I was confiding in my life coach about what I was experiencing and how I was dealing with all of it.

He laughed at me. He chalked it up to paranoia from smoking too much weed.

I knew better. I had always had a better than average connection with God—both before and after the brain tumor.

Once I started practicing more of a holistic lifestyle, this bond had only grown stronger. Marijuana had only helped me to reach that higher plane so much easier.

I believe the practical benefits of regular use of this plant are only starting to be discovered.

As far as I was concerned that day, it was a moot point. I had already decided to follow my own instincts on this one. They had always kept me alive. Thank God I did.

Chapter 23

When my coach failed to support me, I called my husband for advice.

Randi and I have always been confidants of each other. We still talk all the time. He had lived through much of the nightmare in Montana right beside me. He knew not to question my instincts on these kinds of matters.

When Randi heard my entire story, he was concerned for my safety as well. He helped me go online and find a private investigator's firm that was local.

This began a remarkably interesting chain of events in my life. Living through the next several months was quite an adventure. Hold onto your seats while I share the story with you.

First, I met Dick. He was the owner of the private investigator agency. He was an elderly, sweet man. He reminded me of my late Uncle Richard. I felt an immediate kinship with him.

After studying my situation Dick made several recommendations. He wound up selling me a very expensive home security system with cameras and everything. It was very state of the art.

Dick didn't have time to install the system himself or show me how to use it. He was merely there to assess my needs and then sell me the equipment I needed.

After the system was purchased, he introduced me to two other private investigators he knew. They had much more time on their hands and the flexibility to be available to me while we were making the transition to the new system. I would need training on how to use it once they had it all installed.

So, the system was all installed and I was finally "safe." What happened next taught me safety is in the eye of the beholder; literally.

The situation blew up like a keg of gasoline.

Chapter 24

It started when the system was installed—after I had invested a substantial amount of money in the camera system.

It began with the stupid contract Dick drew up for the project.

Someone left the contract with the details about my new camera system laying on the desk in my living room.

I think it was probably me. I was careless about security in those days.

Anyway, when Dick found the contract laying there, he flipped out. He decided that the housekeepers—our number one suspects at the time—had probably found it and read it. To this day, I don't think the housekeepers were on to us at that point.

Dick's solution was to put one of the cameras out in the open so the housekeepers would see it and assume it was the only camera that had been installed. Boy, did this plan backfire on us!

The first day the housekeepers came to work after the system was installed the gig was up.

Even with my limited vision, I was keenly aware Dick's plan had backfired.

The housekeepers were wordlessly gesturing towards the walls and ceilings in my house. I could see them huddling together and whispering. The whole situation made me feel incredibly uneasy. I was alone in the house with them.

I went out on my veranda to smoke some weed.

When I walked back in the door a few minutes later, I was abruptly brought up short.

Bert was suddenly standing right in front of me. On my right side was my large bookshelf that engulfs the entire southern wall of my dining room. Bert's wife wordlessly stepped up close on my left side. My only escape was to turn around and run back out onto the veranda and jump into the pool. I was trapped.

Then Bert confronted me about the camera they could see. He demanded to know the details of the system.

I learned years ago when I was being abused by those people in Montana that I'm not good under pressure. What happened next just proves my point.

I looked up at Bert in fear. I nervously glanced over my shoulder. There was no escape.

I opened my mouth to try to lie to him.

As I fidgeted and tried to shrink away from him, I babbled something about still being in the process of finishing, which we were. We hadn't decided yet how many cameras or where we would install each of them. I continued babbling like a fool and blurted out the general location of the hiding place of the brain for the entire system as I flung my arm in that general direction.

They let me go that day. It was about four days later when I realized my "feelings" of being in danger had been completely legitimate.

Chapter 25

I was awakened by something in my bedroom that night. As I was coming to full consciousness, I became aware someone else was in my bedroom. I was hyperventilating as I sat up and rubbed the sleep from my eyes. The thought *"You were right!"* was cascading through my psyche. I was not happy that I was making this realization when I was in such a vulnerable position.

As I was coming to full awareness, I heard a familiar voice in the vicinity of the foot of my bed. When I recognized the voice my first reaction was to relax, it was my friend Marc. He had come over that night to hang out. He was supposed to be in the guest room at the other end of the house. What was he doing in my bedroom?

I stood up and flipped my light on as Marc was making his way back around the foot of my bed towards my bedroom door. He had to walk right past me to reach his goal.

As he lunged for the doorway, I stepped up behind him, grabbing onto his arms to prevent his escape. I firmly gripped his elbows as I held him still in my doorway.

I was aware something might be wrong with my young blind friend. I wanted to make sure he was aware of the situation.

I calmly but firmly asked him in a clear, loud voice, "Marc, what are you doing in my room?" I repeated the question for his benefit.

He was significantly smaller and weaker than me. He was only a threat to me when I was sound asleep.

At that moment I was suddenly wide awake. I knew something was terribly wrong.

Marc tucked his head and whimpered like a weak animal.

When he did this, I released him.

As he jogged away from my bedroom door towards the other end of the house, the thought occurred to me, *What if he stole something from my room before I awoke and caught him?* I quickly spun around and bounded through my bedroom door in pursuit of him.

I caught him just as he was making his way around the fireplace en route to the guest room.

Once I had my hands on that rat, I wrapped my hands around his neck. I then let my body slide to the floor, my arms and hands draping his entire frame on the way down. I was able to discern from my touch he didn't have anything in his hands or pockets. I released him so he could go on his way back to the guest room where he belonged.

When I got back to my bedroom, I made note of the time. When I got up in the morning, I would take care of this little situation once and for all . . . Or so I thought.

Chapter 26

The next morning I threw Marc out. I didn't listen to his sniveling. I had learned how to do this right when I'd thrown Paul and EQ out a few weeks earlier.

Then I called one of the private investigators. I told her exactly what had happened the night before. She agreed to come over and review the camera footage for me.

She arrived at my house as I was leaving for class that morning. I let her inside so she could review the footage from the cameras while I was gone to school. I knew I wouldn't be able to get a report until I returned home that afternoon.

She met me at the door when I returned from class.

First, she sat me down on the couch. She started the video footage from the day before.

As the tape rolled, she gave me a play-by-play description of Marc's arrival the prior evening. She described the meal and activities we had shared together.

She also noted what time she saw both of us go to our rooms for the night.

Then nothing . . .

Until about thirty minutes before I awoke and caught Marc in my bedroom, that is.

Someone found and disabled the unit at that point. The recording just went dead. It was bone-chilling to watch. It was like the plug being pulled on one's very life.

It was only Marc and me in the house that night. I was sure of this because my security system notified me whenever a door or window was opened.

How and why had Marc found and disabled the brain so easily that night?

Upon my own inspection of the unit, it became apparent to me it could easily be unplugged or disabled in several other ways—even if one were blind. I could have done it myself if I'd had the intention and decent directions on how to locate the box.

Other than me and the private investigators though, the only other people who knew the location were the housekeepers.

Why would they have shared this information with Marc?

As this glaring question hit me, I suddenly recalled the many times over the months when I had overheard Bert engaging various friends of mine in conversation when he was working around my home. This wasn't the first time I'd caught one of these "friends" up to no good in my private quarters. I recalled realizing on one of those occasions that Bert had apparently been exchanging contact information with these friends. I remember how odd I found this.

Perhaps Bert was just really friendly?

This excuse only worked when I wasn't finding said friends sneaking around in my bedroom while I was asleep.

This time I saw huge, red flags everywhere.

The most recent occurrence put the whole situation in a new perspective for me. Marc was just a low life who might be interested in stealing from me; I'd had plenty of "friends" do this to me over time. Who had hired him to cut the wires though? Worse yet . . . why? This was what terrified me the most.

I was suddenly flung into a world in which I was scared of my own shadow.

I couldn't answer my front door without nearly having a coronary.

When I had to get into a Lyft or a DAR to go somewhere, I was terrified of who might be behind the wheel.

I was doing crazy stuff like taking a Lyft to a random location, jumping out of the car, running into a business and then fifteen minutes later exiting from a different door after calling a second Lyft from that place to my actual destination. I was really scared.

I'm telling you, I nearly lost my mind I was so terrified.

The private investigators had a solution.

It just so happened it was a slow time for them. They would give me around the clock protection for a fraction of their normal fees while they "protected" me. Slick had her MMJ (medical marijuana) card. This allowed us a common interest to build a friendship upon.

They also set me up with my first taser.

Wow! What a deal. Companionship *and* protection?

Itchie started picking me up for class each morning. He would meet me at the door when class got out in the afternoon to give me a ride home.

I carried my taser with me everywhere, I was so scared. Slick took the night and weekend shift. She'd sleep in the guest room at the other end of the house.

We spent time in the evenings and on the weekends following the "perps" and spying on them together. It was tons of fun and excellent training for me. I knew this exciting life couldn't last for long—it was just a strange situation I found myself in. I knew I had been made for so much more. I was only starting to realize the complete truth. It was time to get to work.

Chapter 27

One day I took a Lyft. The driver was known to me; he had given me rides previously.

When Edge suggested he might stay at my place for a while I thought he was joking. Then I gave his idea a second thought.

I realized having a pair of "good" eyes around for a while might not be a bad idea. I was trying to figure out a way to get my sense of personal security back. I didn't want to continue paying Itchie and Slick for protection. Maybe a roommate was a good alternative.

So, Edge moved in. Inviting so much diversity into my life turned out to be a good decision. The next several months were amazing.

Edge was a stand-up comedian by trade. His ethnicity was black. The fact he was also gay just took the pressure off us both. We quickly became fast friends.

I remember spa days and shopping trips we shared together. I never did talk him into a full Brazilian at the salon that day!

The first time Edge took me to Dutch Bros, I discovered my love of the blended watermelon rebel.

Returning from a trip to Walmart one day, we were laughing and joking as we walked up the driveway together.

From out of nowhere, Itchie was suddenly standing right between us. He jumped up in Edge's face, snarling at him. He said something like, "I've got my eye on you buddy!"

In the moment this happened I was appalled not only at Itchie's crude display of racism but also by the shock of someone suddenly springing up from out of nowhere like that. Imagine what this was like as a blind woman? I knew I had to do something about Itchie's behavior.

It was later that month I had a brainstorm. Why not take Itchie to Missoula with me when I went there over Labor Day? Maybe having him at my side would help me overcome some of the trauma I always experienced when I'm in Montana. It was worth a try anyway.

We flew to Missoula together. I rented Itchie a hotel room.

When Itchie met my husband, it was instant friendship. Just like two peas in a pod; it was hysterical to see.

Randi had always told me I was his only friend in life. I was thrilled to see he had learned how to move on.

Once we were back in Mesa, I started to ease the protection squad away. I really wanted to get on with my life.

As time went by, Edge started inviting me to go to some of his shows. He was bringing the coolest people over to the house to hang out.

When I left Randi, I joined a predominantly African-American church. I certainly wasn't shy about being surrounded by black folks.

I found myself staying out late at Edge's shows nearly every weekend.

Edge took me so many places I had never been to before. It was an awesome opportunity for a blind woman. I met the most dynamic people at these events.

One night at a club here in Phoenix, I wasn't surprised at the enthusiastic reception Edge and I received when we walked through the doors. Folks at the clubs were always struck when they saw us walk in together.

Edge is an attractive, black man of average height. Imagine people's reactions when he walked into a club followed by a tall, blind, white woman with big hair and a long white cane!

On this particular night, there was another reason for people's strong reactions to my presence. For once, I wasn't the only blind ninja in the house.

I had grown accustomed to being unique, to being the center of attention at the clubs. Who was this interloper stealing my limelight?

I had learned from years of experience how very rare it was to stumble across another blind person when in public. It was like a sighting of bigfoot.

This was why I was so thrilled to meet Charmin that night.

Charmin was not only a U.S. military veteran, he was also another of the charming comedians I met through my association with Edge.

The night I met this inspiring man, he was living in a small, cramped apartment in Phoenix with a bunch of sighted comedians. I knew from experience what Charmin was probably dealing with.

Edge and I took Charmin home with us that night. I just knew I could help him improve his situation.

Once at my home, I started showing Charmin the "blind ropes" of life. I taught him how to simplify his existence so it wouldn't be so damn complicated.

I knew how "helpful" sighted people could be. They tend to make stuff so much more difficult than it needs to be.

I found out Charmin was waiting for a spot to become available at the blind rehab center for veterans in Tucson. I offered to let him stay at my house until a spot became available.

During this time, I went with Charmin to his appointments at the Veterans Affairs offices in Phoenix. I met the most amazing, hospitable people whenever we did anything with the VA.

I came into close contact with many of my friends from the blind school at the VA. Several of the staff members with the school were closely involved with activities at the VA. It was nice to see old friends again. I hope to volunteer at the VA someday.

Charmin's case manager with the VA began arranging transportation for us whenever I had to take him into the VA. I was thrilled the day I was invited to ride with.

It wasn't unusual for people to jump to the conclusion I was Charmin's wife when we were at the VA together. I helped Charmin overcome the early fear and frustration of losing his vision. This tends to build quite a bond between two people. I was flattered the way I was so welcomed at the VA.

Edge and I continued living our lives around Charmin as the days went by. It wasn't a problem at all having Charmin in the house.

Edge and I went out of town all the time for shows. Having Charmin at the house gave us a reliable house sitter who could feed the pets while we were gone.

I remember when Edge and I flew to New York City together. As I walked down the city street that night with the lights shining down on me and the traffic whizzing past, I was amazed that I had made it to the Big Apple!

Just surviving my childhood had been a struggle. I never imagined I'd make it so far in life.

One day as Edge and I were driving back from a show out of town, we were discussing our crazy transportation situation.

As a Lyft driver, he was paying something like $149 per week to rent his car from the company. I was paying Lyft $700-$800 per month for unlimited transportation. We realized we could probably do better if we teamed up.

I remember it was Halloween, the day Edge and I bought our car together. What a nightmare that turned out to be.

Chapter 28

We pulled into a random car lot as we rolled into town. We wound up deciding on a beautiful blue four-door car. Edge and I have the same favorite color. It was a very sexy ride.

Everything was fine until I finished signing the final paperwork tying my name to the car loan with Edge.

As I turned to the salesman, I held out my hand to him, requesting a key to the car I had just paid for.

My blood froze when he just laughed at me in reply. When I turned to Edge for support, I received the same response.

I knew I was in deep trouble. I hadn't been treated with such unprofessionalism and disdain since I'd dissolved that damn guardianship in Montana.

Randi had always made sure I had full access to everything, especially when I was paying the bills. I couldn't believe I'd allowed myself to fall into *another* legal trap. I was utterly horrified as I left the car lot with Edge that evening. I knew he had me by the short hairs and there was nothing I could do about it now.

Chapter 29

Charmin eventually moved on to the rehab center in Tucson. He kept in close contact with me so I knew he was well. Life went on for Edge and me.

That December Edge and I flew to Hawaii for a vacation. I paid for the plane tickets. We were going to be staying on base with a married couple who were friends of his so our lodging and most of our food would be taken care of.

On our way to L.A. to catch our flight to Honolulu, we got into an argument about the car. Who didn't see that one coming?

It ended with Edge proclaiming he would simply move out when we got home.

By the time we landed in Honolulu the next morning, Edge and I were barely speaking to each other. The situation only got worse as the days went by.

Chance was a wonderful host. I usually saw him in the early mornings when he was up getting ready for work. After he left the house, I was on my own for the rest of the day. I realized by day two those early mornings with Chance would be my only opportunity to get access to food, fresh water and information.

Edge and Chance's wife Delilah made it clear they had their own plans together each day that didn't include me. I wasn't welcome to accompany them.

I spent my days wandering out onto the beach alone, looking for something to do. I kept getting lost out on the beach when I walked too far down towards the shore.

One day when I was out walking on the beach I wound up in deep sand. I could hardly walk. I became very dehydrated in the hot sun that day.

I was finally able to locate a stranger on the beach who helped me find my way back up to the proper beach house that day. It scared me so bad I decided I better just stay in the house after that.

Life in the house wasn't a bed of roses either. Delilah convinced Edge I was a horrible racist. It was ridiculous.

Edge and I had done so much together, how had he just forgotten our friendship? I was really confused about what happened.

I had gone from friend to public enemy number one as far as my "buddy" was concerned. The whole thing made my head spin.

It really pissed me off, the way this stupid broad was messing up our friendship with her petty, jealous games.

One day as Edge and I passed in the narrow hallway, he decided to confront me about the situation.

He demanded to know if I wanted him to move out of the house when we got home.

What was I supposed to say? *He* was the one who had brought up the subject in the first place that day. He was the only one who could take his words back. I couldn't just order him to stay at my home.

I hesitated, searching for words that would help my friend understand where I was coming from. He clearly didn't trust me anymore.

I finally replied, "I never said I wanted you to move out."

I was shocked when he hissed at me in a low whisper, "If you want me out of your house, you're going to have to take legal action. I've established residency in your house!"

Chapter 30

*W*TF? I think my head spun around I was so shocked. I had a miserable squatter in my house!

Up until that moment, I honestly thought we'd get this whole misunderstanding straightened out once we were back home together. How could we ever make it work now?

I was suddenly gripped with terror. Just who was this man? I realized I didn't know him as well as I thought. Was I safe?

As soon as I was able to find a semi-private spot in the house where I could use my phone without it being overheard, I quickly crafted a text to Dick. I told him to the best of my knowledge where I was and with whom. I advised him I was concerned about my safety. If I didn't turn up in Mesa when I was supposed to, they would know where to start looking. Then I hit send.

I went into survival mode after that. My only concern was maintaining my worldly existence until I could get off of that island.

This meant dodging Edge's attempts to draw me into a verbal argument so he and Delilah could really have a good time at my expense.

To this day, I'm sick at the way Delilah screwed up our friendship with her petty, jealous bullshit.

I was the best friend I could be to Edge and asked only the same respect and honesty in return.

Too bad he wasn't man enough to even meet me halfway.

On our way home, when we landed in L.A., we hit the ground running. I knew Edge would probably flee as soon as possible. Like most people, he can't handle confrontation.

As we pulled into the driveway, I already knew his buddy Jude was on his way from Houston to my house. I was sure Edge had called Jude to run interference for him while he slipped away.

I watched the whole thing unfold right in front of me, completely helpless to do anything about it. I was shocked at how completely powerless I wound up in the whole situation.

Not having a key to the car prevented me from taking possession of it before Edge could take off with it. That damn salesman and his crappy attitude really screwed me in the end.

I knew the day Jude pulled into town his only purpose was to distract me while Edge made his exit. It was so smooth—the way they orchestrated it.

The day Edge took off with the car I knew I was totally fucked. I never saw Edge and that beautiful, blue car again.

Many of the comedians I met through Edge stepped forward in the coming days to express they felt Edge had done me wrong. They wanted me to know they were still my friends. I really appreciated their moral support. I was feeling really used and taken advantage of at that point.

I lived a nightmare after that. The car lot kept calling me until they finally found Edge and repossessed the car.

I received bills for months from various states where Edge had racked up tolls on toll roads and didn't bother to take care of them himself. The whole experience was horrible.

I learned a couple of important things about my friend Edge in the short time I was associated with him. First, he is a royal asshole. I witnessed him going out of his way to be as big of a jerk as he could to people. Second, he is a scoundrel who doesn't recognize untraceable, silver bullion when he has it right in his grubby mitts!

Chapter 31

I was suddenly needed again when Charmin was struck by a pickup truck as he was crossing the street.

He called me from his hospital bed in Tucson, barely able to speak. My heart filled with pain as my friend struggled to tell me about his experiences.

Apparently, some redneck in a pickup truck just blew through a red light, driving right through the crosswalk and over my friend—the blind vet who was using it at the time. This happened right in front of the training center for blind vets in Tucson.

My friend was convinced the guy intentionally tried to kill him because he was black. It tore my heart out . . . the idea someone might have intentionally tried to murder my friend.

As a result of being struck by the moving vehicle, Charmin suffered some very serious injuries. His left leg was broken. He was in a neck brace for a while. His sternum was fractured in multiple places and his right arm was all messed up.

As I became aware of the extent of Charmin's injuries, I realized he would need my support in his recovery.

As the days went by, I became aware Charmin was preparing to be discharged from the hospital. Through my conversations with him, I learned that several "friends" and extended family members were applying pressure on him to come to their homes when he got out of the hospital.

I knew Charmin's wife and children lived somewhere far away. He had nowhere to go nearby where he would be safe while he recovered and regained his strength.

At the time Charmin was expecting a substantial settlement from the VA for his GI benefits. He was also banking on a financial settlement from the incident where he was hit by the pickup.

He had made these two facts known around. People were coming out of the woodwork—lining up to start using him as soon as they could. I knew I had to help my friend avoid getting into such a bad situation.

I suggested to Charmin he could come back to my house when he was discharged from the hospital. He could recover in a supportive, peaceful environment while he regained his strength. I reminded him I had never asked him for any financial compensation when he stayed with me.

I tried to help Charmin understand how important it was to not let himself get into a situation where he would have limited choices.

When I met him a few months before, I worked hard to show him he could live on his own terms even though he was blind.

Suddenly, I had to teach him the same about his new situation before someone else convinced him he needed them.

I helped Charmin make arrangements to have himself transported back to my home upon his release from the hospital.

He was on crutches and brought a walker when he arrived here. There was no way he could have gone back to that upstairs apartment in Phoenix to recover.

His nephew installed a modified shower head in my shower stall for him to use. I purchased a shower chair for his benefit as well. He was able to use the support bars I had installed for my own safety for his use while he showered.

I found the modifications I made to my home for my mother-in-law's use following her surgery made it very easy to convert the rest of the house for Charmin's comfort during his recovery.

I really felt like God had been teaching me for years what I needed to know to help this man.

As the days went by Charmin was rapidly getting more mobile around the house. We really made it work.

I was able to be home with him except for my hours spent in class. I spent time teaching him what I had learned in my own experience about recovering from major physical injuries.

On February 3rd that spring, one of my little sisters from Montana moved in with me.

I had been trying to get Ami here since I first moved to Mesa. I found it quite significant the first morning she opened her eyes in Arizona was her birthday.

Can anyone say . . . all in God's perfect timing?

If you are one of those people who insist on denying His divine influence in your life, you certainly are a fool.

Everything that has happened in my life over all these decades, as I've done my best to walk a path of faithfulness despite my circumstances, is proof to me that He really does exist.

I have realized He has a hand in our daily lives.

Learning to align my steps with His will for my life has enabled me to walk in daily victory.

Regardless, that day the life coach in me latched on to the idea of new life in our Lord for my little sister's sake.

When Ami and her little dog boarded the plane in Missoula that morning it was blizzarding outside.

A couple of hours later when their direct flight landed in Arizona they walked out into a sunny, beautiful, spring afternoon.

The contrast was striking. For my little sister and her dog, it must have been like waking up in Oz next to Dorothy and *her* dog Toto.

The very first morning Ami and her dog Duke were here, I woke them up early. I saw no point in changing my schedule to accommodate them; I knew what I had to do.

Princess and I took them on a walk around the neighborhood. This started a habit of regular daily exercise for them both.

My sister was fascinated by what she was seeing in nature when she went out walking. She was coming home all the time excited to share her new discoveries with me. It was awesome!

My little sister had extensive experience as a CNA. She voluntarily chipped in on Charmin's care. It was amazing how much happier Charmin was after she arrived.

I had always set up access to food, water, medications and any other resources he would need before I left for class. Having my sister around to see to his every whim while I was out really made his world a wonderful place.

Time went by. Charmin started going out with these two people who just showed up at the door one day. I didn't ask Charmin any questions about who they were or why they were taking him out.

He was already gone one day when my sister and I finally had a chance to discuss the situation.

Apparently, as time passed and Charmin came home from more of these outings with these two people, he had been expressing ever-growing discontent with his circumstances living in my home. There wasn't much more I could do for Charmin at that point. I had already been supporting him for months with no help from any of his friends or family.

When Charmin found out I had no more freebies to offer, he just moved out of my home and in with those two people who had been taking him out. I tried not to take it personally when he blocked my phone number so I couldn't call to say hello.

It was about a week after he was gone when I heard my sister crying out in distress from her bedroom on the other end of the house.

I ran across the house to see what was wrong.

As I arrived at her bedroom door, it sounded like she was hyperventilating she was so upset.

She had discovered her private collection of unique and personally acquired souvenirs had been stolen!

The collection consisted of news clippings, cards, photos and various other collectibles memorializing some of the most important people and significant events in my little sister's life. Several pieces had been given to her by her late father. The collection also contained a few items I had given her over the years. My little sister was devastated.

I remember the day she took her prized possession out of her drawer, sharing it with Charmin and me. That day she told us how much it meant to her and how she had come to possess some of the items. There were cherished memories connected to each of them.

I knew when she estimated the collection's value somewhere north of $35,000, she was thinking of sentimental value.

Charmin took her seriously and obviously hoped to make bank when he sold the stolen items.

As my sister cried about her loss, I began to tell her what I knew about Charmin's family.

I described his brave, young wife whom he had abandoned. I told her about his precious children; a boy and a girl.

She jumped to the conclusion Charmin had stolen the cards to give to his son.

The idea of her beloved treasures bringing joy to such a child gave her great solace.

I struggled with the idea of telling my sister what I suspected Charmin's actual motives had been. I was sure his only intentions had been selfish. Thieves never think of others.

I was mortified. I had introduced my sister to Charmin and allowed her to blindly trust this man. I was so hurt, not only for my little sister's sake but for myself as well.

We had given all our energies and love towards Charmin's care and recovery for months. I had been so devoted to his success that he started referring to me as his "guardian angel."

This was how he repaid us?

The bum actually confronted me about it via a public thread on Facebook a few days later. He played dumb to the whole situation.

I wasn't having any of it; I called him out for the scum he was. He quickly blocked me on Facebook as well.

I wasn't shocked. He had already proven himself to be a coward and a cheat.

Life had to go on.

Chapter 32

That was the spring I wrapped up my training at the blind school. I was learning some interesting stuff about what I was capable of when I advocate for myself. It seemed like the more I challenged the status quo, the more I was finding the status quo wasn't necessarily the best way to look at life.

As I completed my training, I realized it was time to start looking at the future from a new perspective.

I was working on this manuscript during that period of time. I was reviewing what I had already written on the way to continuing my project. I was searching for a way to inject some of God's power into my life as I embarked on my future endeavors.

One day as I was editing, I was inspired to write a challenge to God Himself right there in my manuscript. So I did.

That is the strange passage at the end of Chapter 1 in this book you are currently holding in your hands.

By writing these words I was calling God out, challenging Him to fulfill His promises. As far as I could tell, He owed me big time for my faithfulness all these years. I had been more than patient.

When I came asking, He delivered in a big way. What happened in the coming months made my head spin.

By writing these words, I was working with multiple spiritual concepts. Let me see if I can explain some of them to you.

The first and most important principle is the power to create which we possess in our own words. This includes our spoken and written thoughts, our self-talk in our minds, words others say to or about us and everything we hear and read in our world every day through our media, etc.

This is the food our brains and souls have been receiving.

If it's all destructive and malignant in nature, what then? How can a human soul be expected to thrive under conditions such as those?

This isn't just *my* idea. We are told straight out in Proverbs that we have the power of life and death in our tongues. Why aren't we using it to heal ourselves?

It was only after I learned to view my situation from His perspective that I came to understand these valuable scriptural truths. I have been walking in His power and authority ever since.

If you learn to walk in faith, you too can claim and manifest similar miracles in your own life.

Another important spiritual concept that has gotten me through is that of God's timeline. He doesn't operate under the same time constraints as we do. The Bible says a day is as a thousand years and a thousand years is as a day when it comes to His timeline. He is the author of all eternity.

I found I was able to hyper magnify any results I'm trying to achieve in life when viewing them through this prism filled with His power.

Honestly, I had God on my side from day one. My parents and their sleazy lawyers never had a chance when they schemed against me.

He had begun the healing process when He first created me. I knew all along He would eventually make me whole again.

I continued to claim God's promised healing all those years while my parents, their greedy lawyers and all those stupid doctors argued against me.

Now that I've reached the summit of this mountain, I like the view from up here. It's much nicer than the view from within that hopeless pit I was shoved into when I first awoke.

There are so many foundational principals I've adopted over the years to solidify His presence and power in my daily life.

Chapter 33

*W*hen I was in my early twenties, I realized my biggest problem was this "gotcha game" everyone had been playing on me since I woke up. Everybody compared me and my shortcomings to themselves when they met me. I was always found to be lacking at that point. I just couldn't keep up when compared to the average yogi.

It was only after I started viewing my own opinion of myself and God's opinion of me as the only ones that mattered that I started succeeding in life. This was because I was my own worst critic and God was my biggest fan.

Abuse a person such as this for years and you wind up with a freedom fighter who doesn't know when to give up and die.

That was the relentless creature my parents and their lawyers found themselves battling all those years.

This is the same woman who now owns and operates Blue Butterfly Enterprises LLC.

They better look out now! I'm only getting started.

I have at least three more big projects left to complete before I leave this world.

I can't believe the momentum I have these days. It's incredible! I'm making stuff happen in my life. Check this out. (This kind of stuff happens to me all the time . . .)

One day I climbed into a Veyo with Ami to go to an appointment.

I turned to the driver, engaging him in friendly conversation.

Understanding the situation of many of these private drivers, I asked him what he did in "real life."

When he told me he was a filmmaker by trade, I saw my opportunity. God had placed it right there before me. I went for it.

I informed the driver I had written a book that needed to be made into a movie for the whole world to see.

That day I didn't do any more than just be a friendly person and believe in myself.

I remember months later when Gino and I were reflecting back upon our initial meeting. He pointed out how he heard those words from well-meaning people every day. It was several days later when my sister handed him a copy of my book to take home and read.

I was in Las Vegas at the NFB convention when he called me to discuss the possibility of helping me produce my movie.

Now, the only reason I had my story in a format to share with Gino when God finally brought him to me in the first place was because I had stepped out in faith and obedience in 2013 and published my story.

The process of writing and publishing that first book was a painful and arduous experience. I accomplished it though.

I had always known I had to write that first book—if only to make what my family and I had to go through all those years ago when I was a kid really count for something. I didn't want all our suffering to have been in vain.

Another reason I wrote that first book was because I was angry about all the bullshit those lawyers and doctors had written about me while silencing me. I felt someone needed to write the truth about everything I had experienced—straight from the horse's mouth—so to speak.

I was so bitter after everything they had stolen from me.

I had years to plot my revenge while I was forced to sit back and watch them use my money to plot against me.

All those years I dreamt of the day when I would be able to turn the tables on those crooked, greedy lawyers. I couldn't just let them get away with stealing my very liberty from me.

You better believe; they have created a formidable opponent when they abused this woman. I won't stop until the day I die. Why would I? Proving I'm really alive is my greatest revenge on those ignorant people.

I am the "measuring life" after all. It's about time I get *my* own yard-stick out.

Chapter 34

When I got home from the convention, it was time to get to work. That initial meeting with Gino felt like a dream. I couldn't believe God had brought me my cameraman.

I decided in high school I needed to write my story someday. I could see the writing on the wall even back then. I knew my mother and her lawyers were scheming against me. I prayed I would survive their trap, whatever it turned out to be.

I expected to die in an "accident" before I managed to escape from them.

The idea of making that first book into a movie—if I managed to survive to write it in the first place—felt like a very distant, fanciful pipe dream when I first conceived of it as a helpless teenaged girl.

The day I finally met Gino, it felt like my birthday. I was receiving a long-awaited gift from above.

I had been looking for inspiration since I finished my life coaching training. He couldn't have been more obvious about His leading if He'd had me swallowed by a big fish and then spit out in Hollywood.

How does a blind life coach find an award-winning filmmaker to help her produce her movie?

God delivers one up for her to use of course. At least, this has been my experience.

I'm not kidding. Check this out.

First and foremost, in this tale is this important fact. God directed not only my steps but Gino's as well to manipulate several events in our individual lives. So when we finally met that beautiful summer day, we were both in a perfect position to work together.

It was literally a case of recognizing His call and answering it. That's all we did. He blessed us as a result.

The first thing we did was discuss the basics. Gino was taken aback when I already knew the name of my new company.

Blue Butterfly Enterprises is significant to me.

Blue has always been my favorite color. The butterfly has become a symbol for who I am; that is a creature who is always changing and developing into a newer, stronger and more beautiful version of itself. I chose the word enterprises in that moment because to me this word speaks of excitement and big things to come. It is also a broad term that allows me to be flexible with what I'm working on while still being true to what the purpose of BBE is. (Remember what I said about the power of our words?)

Gino encouraged me to start composing blogs to post on a new website. I was also called upon to develop show ideas for Becca's World, the name of my new YouTube channel.

(I have to admit, I had never been on YouTube before this. I had no idea what a "blog" was either.)

Our motive with the YouTube channel was simple. We wanted to make me better known. Our intention was to make sure our movie would get more traction before we released it—whenever that might be in the distant future. (Making our movie has been a very organic process.)

I quickly realized my YouTube channel was so much more than just an avenue to promote some movie that was yet to be made. Clearly, this was the platform from which I would become the teacher and life coach God had created me to be from the very beginning.

I was so inspired, I felt like the energizer bunny.

I had always wanted to work. I never bought into the idea of sitting on my ass and collecting a paycheck from the government; no matter how large it was or how I had become "entitled" to it.

Once I launched my company, I simply couldn't sit down. There was far too much work to be done. I'm still like a crazy person today, nearly a year later.

Wow! Has it been that long already?

Chapter 35

$\mathscr{I}$ still remember that first blog. It was about my magic cane. I loved writing that first post; I felt like I was able to speak directly to my mother.

I thought about my mom when I filmed my videos as well. This actually helped me to get over any shyness I may otherwise have felt as I was starting the process of learning how to appear on camera on a regular basis.

I simply pretended I was speaking directly and only to my mom when I performed in my videos. I couldn't see the cameras anyway, so it was easy.

My videos became better in topic, substance and quality as time went by.

I was always finding new ideas for diverse shows that were fun and interesting. They were embraced by many viewers. I was so inspired from day one. Building BBE has been an incredible experience.

I have been working on so many fun and inspiring projects since I opened my company. I love being the "boss."

As I produced material for Becca's World, Gino got busy researching and writing the script. It has been a fascinating process learning how to make our 'Oscar Worthy' film.

Crafting a movie that is "based on" your own life story is so much fun. Gino has come up with some ingenious ways to work up the tale to give it a cinematic flair (as if there wasn't enough drama in my story, to begin with.)

In one of the earliest versions of our script, my mother was our star villain. There was a scene in which she could be viewed puffing on a hand-rolled joint in our family's living room. I laughed right out loud the first time Gino read that sketch to me.

Over time, I grew sick at the idea of humiliating my mother with my movie. I have always believed in my heart she was duped into selling her daughter by those greedy lawyers.

In my head, I'm still unable to understand how she could do what she did to her first-born child.

Unfortunately for her, that decision ultimately put her on the losing side in this battle. She should have believed in her daughter a little more.

The day Gino came to work and shared his new vision for our movie with me, I knew he was on the right track.

It was after we got our hands on the audio recordings from the courthouse in Missoula.

I remember how excited Gino and I were when the judge made us sign a form stating I would not take legal action against them before he would release the files to us.

It was while listening to those audio court transcripts Gino realized we needed to center our movie around that two-day trial in 2004.

I knew this was the ticket as soon as Gino suggested it. This was how we would show the world in one fell swoop the problems with these broken guardianship laws.

Then, after we released the movie and got the national conversation started, I would go to Washington, DC with a band of lawyers to talk to congress and take care of this little problem once and for all.

There it is; the purpose for which He made all this happen to me in the first place. After more than 31 years I had finally stumbled upon the fullness of His vision for my life. (Talk about long-suffering!)

I believe it is God's mission for me to take a wrecking ball to these corrupt guardianship laws. I will be the tool in His hand when He frees all Americans from these invisible prisons.

No one can deny the law needs to be changed after they have heard my life's story.

Sadly, I've learned I am just one of many people whose lives have been devastated by one of these legal traps.

Crooked, greedy lawyers all over America are working every day to steal the property and dreams from their "wards."

Someone has to put a stop to it. As the Judds sang, "Why not me?"

Chapter 36

When God brought Gino into my life, He really gave me a boost, both personally and professionally.

Not only did Gino help me establish my company, he also showed me how to relaunch my first book "Because You're Blind" in a much more professional fashion than I had done the first time.

Then he showed me how to get it recorded for Audible.

Making my story accessible to the blind was something I had been wanting to do since I first envisioned writing my book.

I contacted the BARD library in Montana myself and asked them to record it for me.

I was shocked when they refused to help me. I knew my story was unique, even in the world of the blind. Very few people have had their rights as violated as I did.

I have believed for a long time all people—in particular my visually impaired peers—could only benefit from reading my empowering story.

Having a player on my team who possessed not only the knowledge on how to make stuff like this happen but also the same passion as mine, has really helped to springboard me to success in life. God really blessed my efforts when He brought Gino onto my team.

I found success almost immediately with my YouTube channel. Gino and I started looking at it more like a permanent gig for me rather than something fleeting.

When I went blind as a child, my parents decided I no longer had any earning potential.

I had been fighting to disprove this ridiculous notion ever since.

Launching my company was the fulfillment of my plot.

Chapter 37

There were several significant events in my life the year I opened my company.

That August I received a text message from an unidentified number inquiring if I were still looking for a German Shepherd.

Let me explain. My friend Joe had a guide dog who was "retired."

Joe was extremely impatient with this beautiful German Shepherd and seemed like he didn't have time or interest in owning the canine anymore.

I loved the dog and borrowed him all the time to bring to my house, the "dog funhouse."

I asked Joe if I could have the dog since he apparently didn't appreciate the animal anymore.

The selfish jerk refused! I was incensed. His poor dog spent most of his time tied up in the back yard all alone.

At my house, he was allowed to run around and play with the other dogs.

He was also given access to food and water whenever he wanted, instead of when Joe got around to feeding him.

I had been paying for the dog's upkeep for a while because Joe claimed he couldn't afford his vet and grooming bills.

As far as I was concerned, Joe had been taking advantage of me long enough. I felt completely justified when I finally broke off contact with him.

This is why I didn't have his number on my phone anymore.

I knew right away who it was though. Joe was the only person who knew about my quest to find a German Shepherd of my very own.

My feelings were still hurt the day I received his text. He made it all hunky-dory by gifting me my second dog, my Precious.

I believe this was just another move of God in my life . . . Check this out.

When Joe refused to give me his retired guide, I didn't give up. I called around looking for a dog of my own.

The Humane Society didn't have any shepherds. I was told more than once I had to go to a breeder in order to get one.

When I contacted breeders, I found they were too expensive for me. I gave up at that point. I knew God would bring me a German Shepherd if it was His will for me to have one. I simply put my request at His feet and went on with life.

Shortly afterward I received Joe's text message. Was that God? It sure felt like it to me! Don't believe me yet? Keep reading.

How had Joe managed to get his hands on a German Shepherd when I had been unable to find one myself? I knew I was more resourceful than most of my blind friends. No one had ever outdone me. I had a reputation for getting shit accomplished.

It just so happened Joe had a friend who bred German Shepherds. He was able to get one for his small child.

That's another part of this story that I feel proves even more how much God had a hand in this. When Joe realized it wasn't safe for him to have the large, rowdy dog around his small, vulnerable child he gave her to me.

How much more perfect could this have worked out? I have to tell you, I was impressed with God's handiwork!

This is how I know this was God giving me my German Shepherd. He just used Joe to accomplish His task. Precious has been such a great addition to our security squad here at Blue Butterfly Enterprises.

That was also the summer I learned how to use online dating. Imagine that, Blind Becca does POF! (Plenty of Fish.)

I had barely dated anyone, and had no experience doing anything significant online. It was a fascinating experience. (Check out my YouTube channel for a video where I discuss the process if you're interested.)

That October Ami and I traveled to Montana to surprise our elderly grandmother. We snuck in between snowstorms in order to land in our homeland.

We flew into Great Falls late one Friday night. The next morning, we got up early and drove up to the hi-line to surprise Grandma.

We stopped at the local grocery store in Chester to get supplies on our way to Hingham. Walking through the aisles of that store, I was terrified we would run into our mother.

What a relief it was when local acquaintances informed us our notorious mother had moved off of the hi-line two months earlier.

My mother had chosen to go into hiding the very month I launched my company?

I found it hard to believe this was a coincidence.

When Grandma opened her door and realized Ami and I had come to visit her, she was overjoyed, to say the least. Just hearing the happiness in Granny's voice caused my heart to swell with emotion. It had been so long since I'd been in the presence of my sweet Grandma.

I remember so many times over the years as a blind child when I stumbled down that rut-encrusted gravel road and up her driveway to visit her and Grandpa. This lasted until Grandpa got sick with his lung cancer and went to the hospital.

Grandma stopped making her famous homemade doughnuts after we lost Grandpa that fall. She just didn't have the desire once Grandpa wasn't sitting there in his familiar easy chair, puffing on his hand-rolled tobacco smokes and flirting with his bride of so many decades. It was so sad.

That day Ami and I were able to spend the entire day chatting with our Grandma. We ordered lunch from the local café and took it back to Grandma's house so we could continue spending the afternoon with her.

Growing up and then living as an adult in Montana in the shadow of my stepfather and his family was a remarkable experience. Our entire family, including a mutt such as myself, were revered and treated with respect all over Montana because of my dad's reputation. He and my Grandfather were known for being men of integrity and hard work.

I can't tell you how many times over the years people changed their tact when dealing with me if they found out who my stepdad was. I was shocked by how far his reputation extended. I'm so proud to be my stepfather's eldest daughter.

Chapter 38

As fall turned into winter that year—the year BBE was born—I continued working on all my various projects, not the least of which was the completion of this manuscript.

As I made sluggish progress on my book, my YouTube channel exploded in popularity. At the same time, the world around me began to spin out of control.

I'm not sure when it started so I'll just tell you what I know for sure.

That winter the Democrats launched a coup against our dually elected president. They tried to take him and his administration out through all kinds of deceitful and nefarious means. It was horrible to watch as an American citizen.

Well, it was actually a bunch of communists who had been lurking in our government for a long time. They were posing as Democrats to hide their true intentions.

I remember when I was growing up hearing members of my community predict these people were lurking in our government, just waiting to usher in communism when they had the chance. No one knew back then which party these people would eventually emerge from.

We all knew well the evils of Communism; we had been watching what was going on in the Soviet Union on the news every night. We grew up understanding the shortcomings of socialism.

As a child, I found these rumors frightening, to say the least.

As an adult who has been watching the Democrats' disgusting grab for power, I'm just royally pissed off at this point.

They've messed with the wrong American woman this time! You better believe, my country's enemies—both foreign and domestic—have a formidable opponent standing right here.

I love my country and would gladly spend the rest of my life fighting to defend her. I'm already on a mission and have just been handed a very large megaphone in the form of my YouTube channel. Guess what happens next?

Blind Becca becomes a self-styled social justice warrior in her own right.

I've always been a rebel, I guess.

I think it started when I woke up. I had to refuse to accept *their truth* in order to survive. Eventually, the mantra I had been repeating in my mind to empower myself really did become my truth.

I truly believe this is the heart of how I finally defeated all those highly educated and sadly misinformed people in Montana.

I literally believed in myself and what God had said about me until it became my truth. It was kind of like positive thinking on steroids.

I know with this knowledge, I can accomplish whatever I set my mind to in life. So . . . what's next?

Chapter 39

I met Big D. on November 5th, 2019. We initially found each other on POF.

When I set up my POF profile, I selected black male from the menu.

It was crazy that women could just go online and shop for a man as though they were browsing through a catalog looking for a new pair of shoes or something.

I had been trying to "bump into" the perfect guy for years. How had I not known about online dating?

I'm serious. Why do you think I joined that black church when I left Randi in the first place?

I was trying to meet a nice black guy. I realized after a while even though I was surrounded by lots of nice black folks, most of the males were either married or under the age of consent.

Being neither a homewrecker nor a pedophile, I realized I was barking up the wrong tree. Back to the drawing board.

I was thrilled with the POF app for the iPhone. It was so accessible.

You're probably asking yourself exactly what my blind girlfriends wanted to know when I told them about my experience . . . *did I reveal my blindness on my profile?*

The answer is, absolutely not. I never do.

It's not like I attempt to hide my blindness, it just doesn't come up in normal conversation.

There is no "Are you blind or sighted?" on most of these sorts of questionnaires in life.

On an even more important note, if anything, my blindness compliments me. I feel like bringing it up would be akin to bragging. I don't want people's first impression of me to be that I'm conceited.

On the other hand, bringing it up and presenting it as though I were ashamed of it (which I am not), would just serve to put me at a huge disadvantage from the start of any new relationship.

This is why Big D was shocked that night when he opened his door to find me standing there proudly holding my long, white cane.

By then, all he could do was wrap his arms around me and pull me into his embrace, passionately kissing me. We spent the holidays together that year.

Chapter 40

The Democrats promised to deliver an impeachment to the nation for Christmas that year. Their entire production made me and everyone I knew absolutely sick. I laughed my ass off when their stupid plans backfired on them.

It was shortly after Christmas when I remember hearing the words "Wuhan China" for the first time in my life.

We started hearing rumors about something called a "wet market."

As an average American, I was oblivious to what had been happening on the other side of the world.

The news eventually broke the Communist Chinese government had manufactured and then "accidentally" released a deadly virus into the world. They were found to have taken measures to protect their own countrymen while foisting the virus onto the rest of the human race.

That virus eventually came to be known by its most accurate and appropriate title "The Chinese Virus." People all around the world were terror-stricken, to say the least.

There's much more to the story but I'm here today to talk to you about a much more pressing matter than dying from some silly virus. Our very liberties are in jeopardy in this country!

The next several months were like living through an episode of "War of the Worlds."

We were ordered to stay in our homes to avoid spreading the virus to one another. We had to have masks covering our faces to go out in public.

The government told us we couldn't open our businesses or congregate at church or other public gatherings.

There were stories of Democrat lawmakers and other government officials using military-grade helicopters to spy on their citizens to ensure their adherence to the newly established Democratic policies.

As a result of this, the productivity of America ground to a screeching halt.

Honestly, it was like the whole damn nation was locked down under its own giant guardianship. I was spitting mad!

I had only had my constitutional rights for a few years at that point. Now, thanks to the cowardice of my fellows, I was in danger of losing them all over again.

I knew how to stay productive while locked down under a guardianship though. As the rest of the world was forced to sit back and twiddle their thumbs, Gino and I raced full speed ahead on our projects.

I came to realize what my mother meant all those years ago when she described my settlement as "disaster-proof." When the quarantine came down, as everyone else was losing their *asses*, I kept getting my monthly paychecks. This enabled me to continue on with all my projects unabated. Not only have I been able to keep both of my households afloat, I've also been able to keep Gino on the payroll through it all.

Having so much time on my hands these last several months has enabled me to get caught up. I'm literally days from sending this manuscript on to the editor.

It was ridiculous.

There were rumors of wide-spread deaths and chaos not only here in America but all around the world.

The entire earth was terrified and mourning.

I remember in January that year when Iran "accidentally" shot down a Ukrainian passenger jet.

That was the same month the world lost Kobe Bryant, his beautiful, precious daughter and several other innocent people in a tragic helicopter crash.

Thus, were the unusual elements in America as we emerged into the year 2020 A.D. Life in America felt like a roller coaster from day one.

Chapter 41

As the orders were coming down that state-to-state transit would be restricted, my sister and my boyfriend were staying here at my house with me.

I received word a woman I met in Montana in October was fleeing for her life from that wretched state. (You better believe I understood her fear and anxiety.) She was headed for Mesa.

As all of these events were happening, I had just one main concern. Were our supply of food and fresh water adequate to get all of us through if conditions on the ground became desperate?

Growing up in Montana, we were taught to take care of ourselves, not to expect the government to come galloping in at the last minute to save us. The principals I was taught growing up just took over.

Upon inspection of my deep freezer, I realized it was several years old. If it gave out, we would lose our entire stock of frozen meat.

When I was a child, my parents always had two deep freezers if they could get their hands on a second one. They would load them up with venison and other wild meats as well as cuts of beef, chicken, and pork from the local butcher. This was what sustained our family through the long, harsh winters in Montana.

I was really sweating it. They were on backorder everywhere by then.

The freezer I ordered wound up not coming to me until the first week of July that year.

There was a run on the gun stores as well. I was relieved I already had my hunting rifle as well as a few boxes of shells to go along with it. How I longed for a handgun for personal protection though!

When Rita arrived from Montana, she had her two dogs with her. Back in October one of them was sick with a gross infection on the side of its face. She still hadn't gotten the animal treated.

My sister and boyfriend made sure to describe it to me.

I told Rita the dog couldn't come into the house where he might make our dogs sick. There was literally blood and puss oozing from the wound. I didn't want that infection all over the floors in my house where it would be picked up by our feet and spread everywhere. I had to think about biohazards; we already had a badass virus on the way we had to figure out how to contend with.

This created problems with Rita. The chick was really out there.

After a lot of yelling and dramatic shit, she decided to put the dogs in her car she had pulled into our garage. Then she came into the house and ate with us.

For several days she was in and out of the garage, tending to her animals. Over time it became apparent she had pulled her car into the garage because she was hiding from the authorities.

She had my roommates and me convinced for nearly a week that the police had our house surrounded. They were supposedly waiting with guns to shoot her as soon as she emerged. I became concerned they would accidentally shoot one of my roommates or me. It was ridiculous!

Then one cold night Rita made several trips in and out through the door connecting the garage to the house after we had all gone to bed. I got out of bed a couple of times and questioned her about what she was doing. She proved evasive. Eventually, I wound up locking the garage door to keep her from coming back into the house, it was so disruptive to our sleep.

In Montana that would have been a death sentence; she would have frozen to death. In Arizona, it enabled her to really take advantage of us.

I was royally pissed off when I eventually found out what she was up to that night while we were all trying to sleep.

Looking back, all I can do is laugh my ass off at what happened.

After I locked the garage door, I began to feel guilty. I got back out of bed and went to talk to Rita to try to help her figure out what to do.

My understanding was her car battery was dead.

When I opened the garage door, I was met with Rita's mug yelling in my face, "Ladies and gentlemen, this is the lady who is refusing to let me and my dogs in her house!" She added with a vicious snarl, "This is going out live over my YouTube channel!"

Chapter 42

*M*y first thought? *Oh no, you didn't bitch! I've taken on bigger men than you and won.* I wasn't intimidated by a little thug like her.

I realized I was standing there in my nightgown (thank goodness it was appropriate because I hadn't known I was going to be on camera when I opened my garage door that morning).

I am Blind Becca though; creator of Becca's World. I know how to handle any situation.

I opened my arms wide. I announced in a loud, clear voice for the benefit of Rita's YouTube audience, "Ladies and gentlemen, this is the woman who has been hiding in my garage from the police for nearly a week. She has had my family and me living in fear for our very lives."

You better believe it, Rita shut her app in a hurry when I did that.

Then I grabbed my phone and dialed 911.

I told the police dispatcher what was going on in my home. She agreed to send officers to the scene.

When the officers arrived, they ran Rita's name. She didn't have a warrant after all.

They jumped her car so she could get out of our garage.

After Rita was gone and the police had cleared out, we discovered she had stolen a lot of stuff from us.

She cleaned out half of our deep freezer in the garage. (Don't ask me what her plans were for a bunch of frozen meat; she didn't have a freezer to store it in or a kitchen to cook it in.) What a Brainiac!

She stole so much stuff from my roommates and me. We were discovering for weeks afterward various stuff around the house that was missing.

When she sped out of here that day, she had no way to get her car to start again once she eventually turned it off or ran out of gas. Her entire flight made no sense to me. Why would you alienate your only friends like that? She didn't know anyone else here.

I was horrified. What were we going to do now? I had just spent a fortune stocking that freezer.

Chapter 43

Big D and I were fairly new in our relationship when the quarantine came down. It put us in an awkward position.

I was aware he didn't have a place to go that was secure.

I also knew having a man around would help keep my sister and me safe during the quarantine, however long it turned out to be. (We're just now trying to come out of the quarantine as I write this passage.)

Honestly, it was my survival instincts that led me to shack up with Big D initially.

Over time, the three of us became like a family as we fought to survive the quarantine together.

Just before all this happened, I ordered a big smoker grill and a fire pit from Home Depot.

They were delivered just as the lockdowns were being announced.

We were able to have get-togethers with a few friends in the backyard where there was plenty of room for social distancing. It really made the quarantine more bearable for all of us.

Big D is a great cook when it comes to that grill. He makes magic each time he fires it up.

He really loved cooking for all of our friends. We had so many great times together during that wretched lockdown!

I believe the China Virus went through our household in March of that year. As our resident historian, I tried to watch for it and document everything that was going on here on that front.

Ami and I both started running fevers over the two days after we called our sister on her birthday that month. By that weekend, both my sister and boyfriend were violently ill with worse than "normal" flu-like symptoms.

I never did become "sick" in the traditional sense. I only felt a bit more fatigued than usual as my body fought off the fever.

It took between fourteen and seventeen days from the first onset of symptoms before I felt we were all clear of the virus.

I wasn't surprised at the way my body responded.

I have never had a flu shot or any other vaccination not required for school admission. I know I have the immune system of . . . someone who doesn't have to worry about biological threats from crazy Communist dictators, I guess.

A lot of crazy stuff happened in my life during that quarantine. It was during that time I fired my life coach. That's right . . . I fired him!

What happened to cause me to make that decision is irrelevant.

What I found so compelling was what I learned about myself through this experience.

I realized I had become my own best life coach. I didn't need my coach anymore. He literally worked himself out of a job.

My heart grieved constantly for my boys up in Montana from the time they left. I felt guilty for a long time I allowed their father to just take them up there like he did. Maybe I should have put up a fight? It just seemed like the boys needed strong, male guidance—something I wasn't equipped to provide them with when I left their father. So, I let them go.

When this damn virus hit, I realized Montana was probably the safest place in America for my children.

I stopped begging God to bring them back to me after that.

Life went on. The new regulations never did feel "normal" to me.

Then, on Memorial Day... George was murdered.

Chapter 44

George died right on cue; almost as if his gruesome death were a setup. He died at the hands of one of Minneapolis's finest; a police officer.

The horrific act was caught on tape.

I'm glad I couldn't "see" the footage that was splashed across all our screens that spring. Listening to it proved gruesome enough.

There were several things about this murder that set people off.

Overnight what had been peaceful protests of the government's overreach of power became violent riots in the streets of Democrat-led cities across America.

People just went nuts. They went out on the streets and vandalized their neighbor's property.

Many innocent people were injured; some were killed.

When our police tried to render aid, they were attacked and murdered by violent "protestors."

Worst of all, the Democrat lawmakers pretended this wasn't happening to their cities. They sat back and made jokes while their cities burned and their citizens lost their livelihoods to the rioters.

Again, and again while President Trump offered support from the federal government, Democrat governors and mayors refused federal aid while their citizens suffered and died in the streets. It was sickening to watch.

Even a blind woman such as yours truly could see from the news we were under attack from an army that had been trained, equipped and then set upon the American people with an agenda.

Initially, they were known as "Antifa."

This is when our right to own firearms became really important. Who were you going to call when the police were on the run and the potential bad guys were your fellow citizens?

Yourself, your God and your guns are all you have when you find yourself in a situation like that. The Democrats want to take your guns away. Get it?

The murder of George Floyd was a horrible, disgusting crime against humanity that happened to be caught on film.

I'm glad I couldn't "see" the footage as it was splashed across our screens.

Listening to the footage proved gruesome enough.

That wasn't the only murder of an innocent, unarmed black citizen in America that spring. George was just the one who fit the agenda of the radical left.

They needed a shocking crime to set off the domino effect it took to bring about socialism here in America.

This was their big chance to force their illicit political agenda down the gaping throats of the American voters. (The American people have been gagging ever since!)

Around that same time news broke Joe Biden was the presumptuous front runner for the Democratic nomination for president.

Let me tell you, this made me laugh my ass off.

The DNC had stolen the nomination from Bernie Sanders again!

It was the same bogus performance the Democrats had given in 2016 when Hilary was a flop. Now, the shenanigans were starting all over again with Biden.

Then, like all of the Democrat's stupid, underhanded tricks, this scheme also backfired on them.

They wound up with a bumbling old fool on their ticket who only looked worse as the weeks went by.

I was laughing so hard through all of this. Mostly because all four of my misled parents lean left politically. (Oh, to be a fly on their wall!)

Chapter 45

*A*fter everything I learned throughout my life in Montana, I understood the importance of protecting *all* of our rights. It was individuals such as the "common law" citizens who refused to license their automobiles that got me thinking maybe there was strange power in our laws.

I watched the "Freemen" while they had their standoff with the feds over their right to bear arms.

It was far back in the badlands of Montana where the Unabomber plotted and then carried out his gorilla-like attacks on society.

Needless to say, I grew up learning to think like a vigilante.

Then I was dragged into court when I was 20 years old and stripped of my rights.

When I finally had the opportunity to read the Constitution in 2004, I realized almost every one of the protections that are guaranteed to all Americans had been denied me through the administration of that damn guardianship.

This is when I saw red. I knew I had to get even with those fucking lawyers.

They stole my life from me by twisting the law. I simply figured out how to twist it back the other way.

You see, as I pointed out in my previous book, the legal statutes regarding capacity are extremely vague, thus leaving them open to broad interpretation. What isn't unclear is what the Constitution says about our rights as citizens.

Once I changed my perspective, I realized my interpretation of these same laws was just as valid as that of those sleazy lawyers.

I simply shared my interpretation with the judge through my lawyer in court that day.

He knew I was right. I finally had those lawyers by the short hairs in court!

I remember the ruckus across the aisle in court when those sleazy lawyers from the bank realized I had outsmarted them. Laugh my ass off!

This is my point. There is a lot of power in the written word, especially when it's written in a divinely inspired document such as our Constitution.

If you stand on those written laws, no court can legally refuse to give you back your property and all your rights—including that of self-determination.

Now, as my tale draws to a close, there's just one more urgent topic I need to discuss with my readers today.

We are on the very brink of sliding into a communist nightmare.

We have been prepped for months, really years now. Just look at what's been going on here in America.

First, they have destroyed any ability you have to take care of yourself. Then they convinced you that you can't depend on yourself or your fellow man. Finally, they are dragging you into court to strip you of your rights. It's the same thing my parents and the state of Montana did to me in 1997.

This is what the Dems have been doing to us.

Well, they think they have us by the throat and are dragging us up the courthouse steps as we speak. I think they have another thing coming though.

They have grossly underestimated the spirit of the American people and the integrity and commitment of our president, Donald J. Trump and his administration. The big showdown will be in November. I hope to see you at the polls!

Chapter 46

have several projects I'm currently working on here at Blue Butterfly Enterprises. I invite you to contact me if you would like to participate in any of them or just want more information.

You can stay up-to-date on my projects by subscribing to Becca's World on YouTube.

You can also email me at info@bluebutterflyenterprises.com if you'd like to participate.

Some of these projects include:

- Videos on Becca's World that are designed to educate, uplift and inspire individuals.
- Blogs that are designed to share my unique perspective on the world.
- The production of a movie based on my first book "Because You're Blind.".

And finally, my latest project, my Declaration of War on guardianship abuse.

I invite you to subscribe to Becca's World on YouTube and follow my website bluebutterflyenterprises.com if you'd like to get involved.

I have proven with faith in yourself and what God said about you, you can accomplish whatever you set your mind to in life. You are not restrained by your current circumstances. If you can imagine it; it doesn't matter how blind the people are who surround you. You can achieve it if you believe in yourself. Go get 'em tiger!

Facts and findings of Blind Becca:

1. God and the American people put President Trump in the White House.

2. The forces that are trying to overthrow our president—both foreign and domestic—will not succeed in their efforts to undermine our Constitution and republic.

3. The American people will prevail in November and beyond into a new season of prosperity as we continue to move forward despite this stupid virus.

These are my decrees; written this day and given the same power and authority all my words have these days.

As it is written, so be it.

Rebecca S. Meadows,
Founder and CEO of BBE and creator
of Becca's World on YouTube August, 2020 A.D.

About the Author

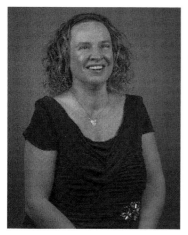

Photo by: The Real McCoy Photography

Rebecca Meadows lives in Mesa Arizona. From her headquarters she manages her company; Blue Butterfly Enterprises LLC.

She is also the host and creator of Becca's World on YouTube.

She is currently working on producing a movie based on her first book "Because You're Blind" and is beginning the process of writing her third book.

Through videos on her YouTube channel and her writings; Ms. Meadows is fulfilling the mission she believes she was called to; to educate the world on how to free themselves from the enslavement of their minds.

Ms. Meadows spends her days working hard on several projects; each designed to help others discover the power they possess to change their own lives.

Made in the USA
Columbia, SC
14 March 2024

32819182R00083